The
Insomnia
Diaries

The
Insomnia
Diaries

How I learned
to sleep again

Miranda Levy
Foreword by Dr Sophie Bostock

aster

First published in Great Britain in 2021 by Aster,
an imprint of Octopus Publishing Group Ltd
Carmelite House
50 Victoria Embankment
London EC4Y 0DZ
www.octopusbooks.co.uk

An Hachette UK Company
www.hachette.co.uk

Some of this material previously appeared in articles Miranda Levy
has written for the *Telegraph*. Discover these and more at
www.telegraph.co.uk/authors/Miranda-Levy

ISBN 978-1-78325-418-7

A CIP catalogue record for this book is available from the British Library.

Publisher: Stephanie Jackson
Editor: Ella Parsons
Art Director: Juliette Norsworthy
Typesetter: Ed Pickford
Production Manager: Caroline Alberti

Printed and bound in the UK.

1 3 5 7 9 10 8 6 4 2

This FSC® label means that materials used for the product
have been responsibly sourced.

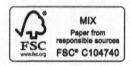

For A and J

Remembering my mum, Wendy Levy,
who I miss very much

Contents

Foreword

by Dr Sophie Bostock

'Can you just give me your top three sleep tips? I've got about 200 words . . .'

My heart sinks. This is the request that everyone working in the field of sleep science dreads. It's not that we don't want to help. We absolutely do. I am a passionate advocate for making evidence-based sleep advice more accessible. I will usually do my best to oblige with the requisite three-, five- or seven-item checklist but I never manage to stick to the word count. The problem is that the longer you've had a sleep problem, the less likely it is that a few generic tips and tricks will hold the key to unlocking better sleep.

Sleep science is not rocket science but the sleep system does have quite a few moving parts. The longer it's been broken, the harder it can be to twist the pieces back into shape.

For this reason, the first time I was introduced to Miranda Levy, when she was a columnist at the *Telegraph*, I have to admit, I was a bit reluctant to pick up the phone. 'This won't take long,' I told myself, stepping out of the library. Forty minutes later, still talking, having done fifteen laps round the car park, I realized I'd left my computer open in the library, my (decaf) coffee had gone cold and I had better get back inside.

Miranda was different. She didn't just want to know what the recommended treatment for insomnia was, she wanted to really understand it. About halfway through the call, I remember her saying, 'Yes, but I've tried that and it doesn't work.'

That's not what journalists usually say. That's what people who have lived with poor sleep for many years say. I took a deep breath and launched into a charm offensive on behalf of the therapeutic approaches that research tells us are most likely to be effective.

If you've battled with a sleep problem for years, it is entirely understandable that you greet every new 'solution' with a healthy dose of cynicism. It can be hard to tell the snake oil from the real McCoy – and, sadly, in the realm of sleep, there is a lot of snake oil out there.

You probably picked up this book thinking – 'Yes, but will it help *me*?'

I can't offer you any guarantees but I can predict that Miranda's story will both intrigue you and teach you something new. If it prevents one person from going down a similar path, it is a valuable book. I hope it will do more than that.

Insomnia is a lonely condition. This isn't simply because you're awake when others are asleep, it's also because of what happens to the sleep-deprived brain.

Our brains evolved to see sleep loss as a warning sign. Our ancestors were more likely to be kept awake by predators than by Netflix, so we tend to respond to short sleep by going into high alert. We get more sensitive to potential foes. For example, we are more likely to interpret neutral faces as threatening and we instinctively want to withdraw from social situations. As the brain channels its energy towards self-defence, we divert resources away from the more rational parts of our decision-making machinery. We get more impulsive and have less control over our emotions.

In the short term, this can mean we react with a short fuse, but in the longer term, we struggle to focus, to learn and remember, to empathize and to make logical, sensible decisions.

We now know that sleep and mental health are inextricably linked. Poor sleepers are at more than twice the risk of future anxiety and depression than good sleepers. While this is no surprise to those who lie awake at night worrying, there is some good news too. Improving sleep will benefit one's mental health.

*

Like most people who feel passionate about sleep science, I fell into it by accident. I've always been curious about what makes people happy. I liked the idea of being a doctor so that I could help people and, since I had a knack for passing exams, they let me into medical school, where I completed a Bachelor's degree. But when, as a fourth-year medical student, we started to encounter real people, unhappy people, I was sadly ill-equipped to cope with the whirlpool of emotions I encountered every day.

I, too, once went to a doctor because I felt unable to cope. I, too, like millions of other people, was prescribed an anti-depressant. I was 22. Talking therapy had a six-month waiting list. I was so terrified by the extensive list of potential side effects that rather than rely on a tablet to solve my career dilemmas, I binned the pills and dropped out of university, in search of some other way.

We didn't learn much about sleep in medical school. (Though sleep deprivation, especially of the alcohol-fuelled variety, was something we were very familiar with.) From what I remember, lectures broke down the body and brain into separate systems: heart and circulation; kidney, lungs and airways; digestion; immune system, and so on. Insomnia was crammed into a 50-minute lecture with sleep apnoea, narcolepsy and restless legs syndrome. It was only really narcolepsy, which involves sudden and sometimes dramatic bouts of sleep onset, which raised a modicum of curiosity from the audience of fledgling medics. Insomnia affects roughly 10 per cent of the UK population; narcolepsy less than 0.1 per cent.

I returned to university a few years later to complete my Ph.D. Still interested in happiness, I decided to investigate why happy people tend to outlive their less optimistic counterparts. This field of 'psychobiology', that investigates the connections between thoughts, behaviour and physiology, was a revelation and not something I had even been aware of at medical school. It turns out that experiencing positive emotions – happiness, contentment – has direct and measurable effects on things like stress hormones, blood pressure and inflammation. So, what can you do to help regulate your emotions and boost the positive ones? The list includes physical activity, a healthy diet and, crucially, sleep.

Sleep makes us feel and look good, helps us learn, improves our concentration, helps us manage our weight, gives us greater self-control, reduces our risk of ill health and is completely free of charge. Despite my basic medical training, I was surprised to discover that at any given time, insomnia means that at least one in ten adults don't have ready access to this panacea. I was even more surprised to discover that the first-line recommended treatment (or first port of call) for insomnia was not, in fact, a pill, but an evidence-based non-drug therapy, cognitive behavioural therapy for insomnia (CBTi), that you will learn more about in this book.

I learned about sleep from Oxford professor and sleep legend Colin Espie. After decades of working as a clinical psychologist in the NHS, Colin and a former patient decided to make CBTi more accessible by creating a digital programme called Sleepio. I spent six years researching and championing the importance of sleep and digital CBTi before becoming an independent sleep evangelist. I've since worked with individuals, companies, healthcare workers, elite athletes, the military and the police to help improve sleep and performance. I think I probably have one of the nicest jobs in the world.

I describe my unconventional career progression in the hope of providing some context for the medical encounters Miranda will tell you about. Medical training has undoubtedly moved on and, fortunately, the availability of talking therapy for mental health conditions on the NHS has dramatically improved. But many doctors in practice now had limited training in sleep science. They may not have been trained in a way that reflects the deep interconnections between the life events, thoughts, behaviours, physical symptoms and support networks which influence our emotional wellbeing, as well as our sleep.

If you go to the doctor with poor sleep today, even the most talented, conscientious and well-meaning GP will struggle to fully evaluate the possible causes and discuss alternative treatment options within a standard eight-minute appointment. Let's face it, prescribing a pill is so much faster. If the patient comes in believing that they need a sleeping pill, it takes a very determined doctor to help them believe in alternatives.

*

When Miranda told me that she was writing this book, I was over the moon for three reasons.

Firstly, because I knew that however dark the subject matter became, Miranda's skill as a storyteller would make it an enjoyable read. It's a rollercoaster.

Secondly, because I am hoping that it reaches you before that critical point when you, or someone you care about, embark on a similar journey. Anyone can be affected by poor sleep. This book will leave you better equipped to avoid common pitfalls and take a shortcut to solutions.

Thirdly, because if you are suffering with poor sleep right now, I hope this book will make you feel less alone. You will be feeling that your challenges are unique, and you're quite right. No one has experienced life as you have. But I hope these pages will help you to realize that there are good reasons for the way you feel, that effective treatment does exist and that, no matter how bad things may seem, there is hope.

Dr Sophie Bostock, 2020

Disclaimer

If you are one of the millions of adults who suffer from insomnia and you are worried about it, speak to your doctor or a qualified medical practitioner.

The author is not a healthcare worker or professional in respect of the issues discussed in the book. The book reflects the author's experience and views on the issues. The author also refers to and interprets the ideas of others. This book is not meant to be used, nor should it be used, to diagnose or treat any medical condition. Any application of the ideas and information contained in this book is at the reader's sole discretion and risk.

PART ONE

Darkness Descends

Year Three

29th June

Eleven forty-seven pm. A door slams as the neighbour's teenage son comes home from the pub. An hour later, the last Tube rumbles past and I thump my pillow over to find a cool spot. I refuse to open the window because of my fear of hearing the first bird of morning, confirmation that the next day is about to start and I have failed, yet again. Failed in my quest to sleep, which one would think is a basic human right.

But I am not a POW whose captors breach the Geneva Convention. No one has stolen my sleep from me. I am not wired up to electrodes, a neon light is not shining in my face all night long. I have blackout blinds and a king-size bed all to myself. My enemies are my brain and a body that has forgotten how to shut down.

I turn over again, pulling the duvet with me until it twists up like a chewed stick of Wrigley's. Where shall I put my thoughts now? I'm too exhausted to read: the words dance in front of my eyes and it's physically tiring even holding up the book. Some nights I write novels in my head, with whole character arcs. But I'm too tired to put pen to paper.

Tonight, I switch on the radio station talkSPORT, where there is an early-hours show featuring two acerbic DJs called 'The Two Mikes'. I have no idea why I listen to this, but something about their banter about things so irrelevant to my own life is comforting and nixes the guilt I feel about 'abandoning' my family, friends and work.

Now it's 3.56am. Just me, and the red numbers on my alarm clock. I see some grey light poking under the blinds. Planes start circling overhead. The milkman delivers his cargo (*who* still gets milk delivered in this day and age?). And now, the kicker: the birds start the dawn chorus that signals the start of another interminable day.

People the world over salute the sun and I fucking hate it.

Five Years Earlier

15th January

8 HOURS A NIGHT, SOMETIMES 9 – OR EVEN 10

My name's Miranda. I like pub quizzes, Earl Grey tea (especially with the school mums after Friday drop-off), a big Bombay and tonic when the magazine goes to press, the Beatles, Maggie O'Farrell novels, hotels, Farrow & Ball paint, my Chloé Bay handbag, talking (a lot) and laughing. Sleeping: going to bed at 9.30pm is a special treat. My two primary-aged children surprise and delight me.

I dislike ignorance and the inappropriate use of apostrophes.

But in the decade to come, I will have no idea what I like or don't like any more. At points, I will barely recognize my reflection, nor my personality. During my Insomnia Crash, and the accompanying Psychiatric Safari, I will lose my job, my home, my looks – even, for a while, my family. My sanity, for sure.

In fact, the only thing I will gain is a stack of weight.

12th May

8 HOURS, 15 MINUTES

It's the night of my 40th birthday. I think I have it pretty much sussed. This weekend, I'll be welcoming 60 friends to a fairy-lit party in the back garden of my north London Victorian terrace.

Trying on my outfit of a poppy-print Joseph dress and purple patent Mary Janes, I reflect on my good fortune. After 16 years of working as a journalist on women's magazines and national newspapers, I have just landed the job as the editor of a top parenting magazine. I have my bright and beautiful kids and a good-looking husband with a professional job.

My wardrobe is full of fashion-forward shoes and handbags. I'm not smug, exactly, but certainly satisfied.

Year One

8th April

8 HOURS, 32 MINUTES

It's my turn to drop the kids at school and I am late. I park near the station and jump on the Tube. This morning we are having a meeting to discuss the testing of nursery products (buggies, car seats, nappies) in advance of our annual magazine awards, which will take place in November. The breast-pump people are being annoying again.

I've been in my job for almost two years now and have grown in confidence. It took time but I have assembled a talented team. We redesigned the magazine and I have twice been shortlisted for a British Society of Magazine Editors Award (Specialist).

I derive great satisfaction from putting together a 'product' (as it's called in these days of platforms, learnings and verbs which have become nouns, and vice versa. Someone actually talked about 'on-boarding' a new member of staff the other day. We all have to choose our hills to die on). It's rewarding to oversee the writers and designers as well as pick up new things about the business side of periodical publishing.

Women's magazines (even the ones about babies) are a glamorous world. Earlier in my career, I worked for several glossies, via a hack through a couple of national tabloid newspapers. One of my main duties is to present the awards at a Park Lane hotel with a celebrity. Before dinner is served, I have to stand up and make a welcome speech, with an autocue, in front of 600 people.

Elsewhere in the job, there are photo shoots and coffee with minor celebrities. Earlier this year, my deputy editor and I went to an event hosted by then-Mayor of London Boris Johnson. We got a bit tipsy and harangued BoJo about the rubbish access for parents with prams around London. 'We want a buggy lane on Oxford Street!' we demanded, jabbing poor, bewildered Boris in the chest.

I feel happy in this publishing company and get on well with my boss. There are hints that I'll be invited to apply for the editorship of a bigger, more mainstream magazine when the incumbent moves on, as seems likely.

After the awards meeting, I have lunch with a contributor in a Soho restaurant, then do some copy editing. I look at the portfolio of a new illustrator we may decide to use. The day speeds by. I rush home, relieve the after-school nanny, bath my kids and put them to bed. I pour myself a glass of Pinot Noir. Then another one. I watch some chat about the upcoming election and check emails on my BlackBerry.

At around 10.30pm, I have a bath, read a bit, then fall asleep immediately. I wake up just before 7am.

16th July

7 HOURS, 22 MINUTES

Two heavy Sainsbury's bags in hand, I navigate the front door. I'm still in gym gear from my Power Plate class. This is my 'magic Friday' routine, when I am not in the office. I'm surprised to see my husband standing in the living room.

My husband and I have been together for 13 years, married for 9, but busy careers and the competitive tiredness caused by 2 children born 20 months apart mean things have started to fracture. (I am 42, he is a couple of years younger.) I know things haven't been great for a while but I distracted myself with my job, friends and family. He starts speaking. I only hear part of what he's saying – such is my discombobulation – but the upshot is this: he wants to call time on our marriage.

I have heard people talking about *Sliding Doors* moments, about rugs being pulled from under them. Now I know what they mean. Nothing will ever be the same again.

I can't recall exactly what happens next but I do have one mission and I won't be swayed from it. Our boy is having his sixth birthday party the next day and I am making a football pitch cake. (The Sainsbury's bags contain roll-out icing, green food colouring and some little goals. I had even sketched out the lines on a piece of paper. This was going to be a major achievement; I am no baker.) Somehow, I manage to sleepwalk through the making of the cake. At some point, I call my best friend and burst into tears, but mostly I am on autopilot.

I go through the usual family bedtime motions and take myself to bed at around 11pm. But I don't fall asleep till after 2am and am awake at around 4.30. I feel myself slipping. I don't want to go 'back there' again.

17th July

2 HOURS, 13 MINUTES

My son has his football party. I don't remember a single thing about it.

18th July

35 MINUTES

'Back there' refers to a six-month experience of insomnia I had several years earlier. A few days before Christmas, I vomited and suddenly started suffering excruciating abdominal pain. Because my kids were nursery age, I assumed it was a gastro bug picked up from them. I was sent home by my GP three days in a row, until I finally pitched up at A&E in the early hours and was diagnosed with a burst appendix.

This led to emergency surgery on Christmas Day, peritonitis and septicaemia. The doctors told me I was lucky to be alive.

While I escaped physically unscathed thanks to the skill of my surgeons, two weeks on a bright, noisy NHS ward hooked up to intravenous antibiotics seriously interfered with my sleep. When I got home to my dark, quiet bedroom, things surprisingly did not improve.

For several months I was incapacitated by insomnia, unable to work as a freelance writer or properly engage with my children, then toddlers. The occasional prescription of sleeping pills helped, but only for a couple of hours a night. My husband stepped up (something for which I will be eternally grateful), although I was still determined to do the best I could as a mummy. But my kisses were half-hearted and I spent the whole day gearing myself up just to put the kids in the bath and read them a story.

The words in the storybooks could have been in Mandarin. Goldilocks, Meg and Mog, Charlie and Lola – they all conspired to mock me as they invariably ended up going to bed.

Eventually, with the support of my husband and an empathetic psychiatrist who put me on a 'subclinical' dose of trazodone – a sedative anti-depressant which I was told can aid sleep in low doses – I started to get better. Almost imperceptibly, I found myself sleeping a bit more every night and gradually got back on my feet again. And for the next four years, things were great: better than great. I got the job as the editor of the parenting magazine, and slept eight, nine, sometimes ten hours a night.

This time around, I don't have the time to heal, nor the support of my husband. I call the consultant who saw me four years earlier but he has retired. Do I really want to start again with a new specialist when all I have done is missed a few nights' sleep?

What is insomnia?

The term 'insomnia' might describe your condition if:

- You have difficulty falling or staying asleep, or your sleep is 'non-restorative' (i.e. you don't feel refreshed in the morning).
- You have this problem even though you have time to sleep and nothing external is keeping you awake.
- You feel upset and impaired while performing tasks the next day (impairment and distress are the big giveaways).

How common is insomnia?

Thirty per cent of adults experience sleep problems, according to researchers, with some estimates putting that figure as high as fifty per cent. One in ten are said to suffer from chronic insomnia.

I think it's safe to say that pretty much everyone has experienced at least a short run of broken nights – and knows how demoralizing even this can be.

Who is most at risk?

Insomnia can get its vindictive hooks into anyone, at any time. But you're more likely to suffer if:

- **You are a woman:** According to one paper, women are 40 per cent more likely to develop insomnia than men. Sleep problems can arise during pregnancy and during the night sweats and hormonal changes of the menopause. Women are also more likely to have the responsibility of looking after young children and elderly parents, as well as going to work. No wonder we are often stressed.

- **You're over 60:** Biological changes can make sleep more difficult as we get older. For example, some older adults experience a shift in circadian rhythm (body clock) that causes them to become sleepy in the early evening and to wake up too early the next day. Certain medical conditions related to age – such as chronic obstructive pulmonary disease (COPD) and Alzheimer's – can also cause insomnia.
- **You suffer from sleep apnoea:** This condition that causes a person to briefly but repeatedly stop breathing can lead to broken nights.
- **You have a physical illness or emotional distress, or you are worried about something.**
- **Your circadian rhythm is all over the place:** Perhaps because you compress your sleep during the week and try to pay off your 'sleep debt' on weekends. Or you work night shifts or are often travelling across time zones. (See page 243 for a long-haul pilot's tips on sleeping despite jet lag.)

What are the different types of insomnia?

Acute insomnia: The short-term, and most common, variety is linked to stress. This could be worries around work – a job interview, for example – or the death of a loved one.

This form of sleeplessness usually resolves within a few weeks. Otherwise known as 'adjustment insomnia', it can also be caused by:

- environmental factors such as noise and light (e.g. not having curtains in your new house; partying neighbours; the tyranny of a new baby)
- sleeping in an unfamiliar bed, such as in a hotel
- physical discomfort, such as post-operative pain, a 'put-out' back, allergies
- some over-the-counter medications. Anadin Extra and Beechams Cold and Flu capsules contain caffeine, which can interfere with sleep. 'Stay-awake' study/party aids, such as Pro Plus and guarana, have high levels of caffeine, and really won't help

Chronic insomnia: A doctor will label your insomnia 'chronic' if you have trouble sleeping for at least three days a week for a period greater than three months. There can be several reasons for this longer-form type of the condition:

- poor 'sleep hygiene' (see page 27)
- physical illness, such as asthma, hyperthyroidism, gastro-oesophageal reflux disease (GORD) and Parkinson's
- sleep-related disorders such as sleep apnoea (see page 178)
- mental health conditions such as depression, anxiety and post-traumatic stress disorder (PTSD). Sleep disturbance is highly prevalent in common mental health 'disorders'. Sleep scientist – and my guru – Dr Sophie Bostock says: 'Stress comes in all different forms. Another way of describing it is "hyper-arousal" or an inability to switch off. You might not even recognize yourself as stressed. But you are always "on"'

- medications such as anti-depressants (see the problem here?) and steroids
- lifestyle factors, e.g. shift work and frequent long-haul travel. Your circadian rhythm guides your sleep–wake cycle, metabolism and body temperature. Disrupt this natural rhythm and you may not be able to sleep when you want to

19th July

O HOURS, O MINUTES

I am upset, exhausted and worried about the future. On Sunday night, I visit P, a 'school mum' friend who is a therapist. We have been confidantes for some time. For ethical reasons, P won't counsel me formally, though she recommends a colleague who might. For now, I stick that in my back pocket.

P says I need to act with 'grace' and 'restraint' towards my now-former partner.

The most important thing is for me to get some sleep, she says, so I can continue to take care of the rest of my life – especially as she knows my history of insomnia.

I wonder about sleeping tablets, which I used briefly and intermittently during my Insomnia Mini-Crash. They did occasionally grab me a few hours here and there. P can't advise me but I resolve to see my GP the next day and ask for some pills.

20th July

O HOURS, O MINUTES

I am dazed with sleeplessness. On the way to work, I stop off at the walk-in service at my local GP practice. I tell the doctor I have had some bad personal news. He is harried, in a rush. Almost without looking up, he grabs his green prescription pad and writes me a two-week prescription for temazepam, an old-fashioned sleeping pill. He then 'ups' my trazodone, the anti-depressant I have been taking in small doses as a sleep aid for the past four years.

I continue my journey to work, grateful and buoyed up to face the day, knowing I'll be getting some sleep that night. At our regular Monday morning catch-up, I tell my boss what is going on: we are friends. She is compassionate, telling me I can have time off for medical appointments or even couple's therapy if I need it (I am committed to trying to save my marriage).

She also says the most important thing is for me to get some sleep.

Your first sleepless stop: your GP

It just so happens that my brother's wife is a GP, and a splendid one at that. S did her very best for me throughout my Insomnia Crash (within professional ethics, of course).

She can't speak for all family doctors but this is what S says *should* happen when you visit your doctor complaining of insomnia:

'Every GP manages insomnia in a different way but I do my best to avoid prescribing sleeping pills. Doctors have long been aware of the risks associated with these drugs, though sadly some bad or overstretched GPs still do prescribe them too quickly.

'For me, it depends on the cause. If someone comes to see me in "acute crisis" – for example, their husband has died the week before – I might write a prescription. Before doing so, I am careful to explain that these pills work fantastically – and that is part of the problem: they are addictive. I'll give the patient seven days' supply, suggesting that they only take three tablets in a week and ideally not on consecutive nights. Then I make a note not to prescribe any more.

'If the patient comes back a fortnight later and isn't any better, I might try amitriptyline, an old-fashioned anti-depressant that has a sedating effect.

'If a person presents with chronic insomnia, I will take a different approach. I'll explore the root of the problem in greater depth. Some patients are suffering from depressive illnesses or have "sleep anxiety". I always discuss sleep hygiene (see page 27), but to be honest, 75 per cent of people have tried most of the tips. Sometimes I'll make a suggestion – to get blackout blinds in a too-bright room for example. Or to give up dark chocolate because it's surprisingly high in caffeine.

'But for those who've been suffering with sleeplessness for a while, sleep hygiene probably won't work. In fact, trying something unusual, like changing your bedtime routine – to stop watching TV, for example – might make matters worse.

'All UK practices have access to talking therapy. My area has a programme called "Let's Talk Wellbeing", but this isn't especially for insomnia and I know that patients have had variable experiences with it.

'If I do decide to prescribe a drug, it would probably be zopiclone (see page 31) at the lowest dose. As mentioned above, I tend to only give a seven-day supply; some of my colleagues give fourteen. I can't remember the last time I prescribed temazepam.

'On the other hand, I do occasionally prescribe diazepam (or Valium, which, as a benzodiazepine, is a "cousin" of temazepam). There are two reasons for this. The first is if a patient is presenting with severe back pain. The second is if he or she has "agitated depression", characterized by restlessness and unbearable anxiety. The first line of anti-depressant treatment for this is a class of drugs called selective serotonin reuptake inhibitors (SSRIs) and these can make people feel worse, initially.

'If I'm prescribing diazepam, it will be in a low dose for two weeks, up to three times a day.

'If someone with insomnia comes back repeatedly, I'll start to question whether they are depressed and consider an anti-depressant medication. From the second visit onwards, I'll be asking about their mood: whether they feel low or hopeless. I'll use diagnostic tools provided by the NHS.

'As far as anti-depressants go, the "gold standard" is an SSRI, such as citalopram or sertraline. I give these drugs in 90 per cent of cases; in the others, I'll prescribe a pill called mirtazapine. If there's no improvement in eight weeks, I'll increase the dose. A month after that, I try an alternative SSRI. If there is still no improvement then I may add in mirtazapine to the SSRI, so that the patient is taking two drugs. In my experience, this can be effective.

'If the situation continues unabated for five or six months – and has turned into a mood disorder that I'm unable to treat – I'll refer the patient to a psychiatrist. This is rare, however – I think I've only referred one person in the last two years.'

21st July

0 HOURS, 0 MINUTES

I recall talk of something called 'sleep hygiene' and go online for tips on how to have a 'clean' night's sleep. Here's what comes up:

Ensure you get enough natural light. Exposure to sunlight during the day as well as darkness at night helps to maintain a healthy sleep–wake cycle.

Exercise regularly. As little as ten minutes of aerobic exercise, such as walking or cycling, can drastically improve sleep quality. However, strenuous workouts close to bedtime can promote adrenaline and leave you feeling 'wired'.

Limit daytime naps. There is conflicting advice on naps. Some experts think you shouldn't have them at all, others that you shouldn't snooze within six hours of bedtime or for longer than twenty minutes. The consensus, however, is that daytime sleeping should be limited.

Establish a regular relaxing bedtime routine. A regular nightly routine helps the body recognize bedtime. This could include having a warm shower or a bath. (A University of Texas research paper referred to having a bath as 'water-based passive body heating'. Hilarious.)

When possible, try to avoid emotionally upsetting conversations and activities before sleep. (Such as the *News at Ten*, when the telly is full of depressing stories.)

Steer clear of rich or heavy food. Fatty, fried or spicy dishes can trigger indigestion in some people. When eaten close to bedtime, this can lead to sleep-disrupting heartburn.

Avoid stimulants such as caffeine, alcohol and nicotine close to bedtime. When it comes to alcohol, moderation is prissily key. While booze is well known to help you fall asleep more quickly, drinking close to bedtime can disrupt sleep in the second half of the night as your body begins to process the alcohol.

Make sure your sleep environment is conducive. Your mattress and pillows should be comfortable and the coverings should ideally be made of natural fibres. Your bedroom should be cool – between 18 and 21°C. 'Blue light' from lamps, mobiles and TV screens blocks the production of the sleep hormone melatonin, and can make it difficult to fall asleep, so turn them off an hour before bed. (Good luck with that one.)

Use blackout blinds, eye shades, ear plugs, humidifiers, fans and other devices. These can improve your sleep environment by making it darker, quieter and more relaxing.

Sleeping pills, anti-depressants and other 'sleep aids'

'Sleeping pills' and anti-depressants are not the same thing.

Sleeping pills (also known as 'hypnotics') are supposed to be a short-term solution, whereas anti-depressants are said to improve mood for the longer term.

Benzodiazepines

The most notorious of the hypnotics are the benzodiazepines – 'benzos' for short – drugs that end in the suffix 'pam'. They are sedatives that work by increasing the effect of a brain chemical called GABA (gamma-Aminobutyric acid), which makes you calmer and sleepier.

Benzos are ideally avoided these days because they carry a long-acknowledged risk of dependency/addiction.

At the time I sought advice from my GP, guidelines from the National Institute for Health and Care Excellence (NICE) were that benzodiazepine hypnotics could be used but only if insomnia was severe, disabling or causing the person extreme distress. And then at the lowest possible dose, for a maximum of four weeks, intermittently if possible. These days, benzos are no longer 'routinely recommended' for the treatment of insomnia. Anecdotally, however, I hear they are still often dished out like peanuts at the pub.

Different benzos have different 'half lives' (the length of time they are active in the body). Sleeping pills have shorter half lives; tranquillizers take longer to leave your system. Pills with shorter half lives are said to be more addictive.

Benzos include:

Temazepam (a sleeping pill which is barely prescribed any more) and **diazepam** (a.k.a. Valium, or 'mother's little helper'). Diazepam was scandalously overprescribed in the 1960s.

Lorazepam is often used in hospital settings and Librium (**chlordiazepoxide**) to help with alcohol withdrawal.

The infamous date-rape drug Rohypnol (**flunitrazepam**) is also a benzo.

Clonazepam (brand name Rivotril) is given for anti-anxiety and was my 'entry-level' drug.

As we will see, I had *terrible* problems with benzos.

Side effects can include:

- drowsiness
- light-headedness
- confusion
- muscle weakness
- memory problems
- issues with withdrawal and dependency

'Z-drugs'

Rather than prescribing a benzo, most modern GPs will give you a Z-drug (usually zopiclone in the UK) for insomnia. The Z-drugs were developed to find an effective but less addictive solution to insomnia than benzos and many doctors still believe they are less habit-forming.

'Z-drugs' include **zopiclone** (Zimovane) and **zolpidem** (Stilnoct). Don't you love the way the marketing experts/people who name drugs promise you something lovely? (In America, zolpidem is known as Ambien, which brings to mind a zoned-out rave in Goa.)

In 2015, NICE said: 'Guidance states that there is no compelling evidence of a clinically useful difference between the "Z-drugs" and shorter-acting benzodiazepine hypnotics from the point of view of their effectiveness, adverse effects, or potential for dependence or abuse.'

In other words, they are just as bad.

When I was first prescribed Z-drugs, the treatment guidelines were the same as those for benzos: a maximum of four weeks and only to be taken intermittently. But, in January 2020, the guidance changed. NICE now advises that hypnotics should be prescribed for short-term (two to four weeks) use only when non-drug measures have failed and insomnia is severe, disabling or causing extreme distress.

At the time of writing, I have been on and off them for ten years.

The side effects are similar to benzos. According to Dr Bostock, both carry increased 'risk of death'. Cheerful.

Other sleep drugs

Antihistamines: Primarily used for treating hay fever and other allergies, antihistamines can cause drowsiness, hence they are also used for short-term sleeping problems. You buy them over the counter. Nytol, for example, contains the antihistamine diphenhydramine and Night Nurse contains promethazine.

Some psychiatrists prescribe **promethazine** (a.k.a. Phenergan) for insomnia instead of benzos. This does apparently work for some but for those who need serious sedation (i.e. me) antihistamines don't even touch the sides. Though in my case, maybe some of that was psychological – I remember being given Phenergan for travel sickness as a child and therefore didn't take it very seriously.

Side effects can include:

- drowsiness and reduced coordination, reaction speed and judgement, so they are not recommended for anyone driving or operating 'heavy machinery'
- dry mouth
- blurred vision
- difficulty weeing (apparently)

Melatonin: A hormone found naturally in the body, this regulates the circadian rhythm. The brain manufactures more melatonin at night, making a person sleepy. Daylight decreases melatonin production, hence you wake up.

For a while now, drugs companies have been making melatonin synthetically in a laboratory, most commonly available in pill form. Synthetic melatonin is often used to adjust the sleep–wake cycle – e.g. for jet lag and for people who do shift work – but isn't actually indicated for insomnia.

In America, you can buy melatonin at a chemist – you often see it at airports over there. In the United States, over-the-counter melatonin use more than doubled between 2007 and 2012. In 2012, a reported 3.1 million individuals (1.3 per cent of the population) were taking the drug.

Only one melatonin product – Circadin – is licensed for use in the UK and you have to get it on prescription because doctors over here feel there is a risk of dependency. Melatonin is actually only licensed for adults aged 55 or over and for a maximum of 13 weeks, though some psychiatrists do use it for younger people.

Side effects can include:

- headaches
- dizziness
- nausea
- drowsiness

Anti-depressants

Anti-depressants are said to work by boosting or prolonging the activity of certain brain chemicals, such as serotonin and noradrenalin – 'neurotransmitters' which affect mood. At least, this is what I was told and this message is still out there all over the Internet and in doctors' surgeries. Though anti-depressants do appear to help some people, the baffling truth is that not even the experts are completely sure how they work. An increasing body of work suggests much of the effect may be placebo. **(Though DO NOT come off your anti-depressants without speaking to a doctor.)**

There used to be a theory that they correct a 'chemical imbalance' in the brain but that was disproved in the early 2000s. Several doctors I encountered on my Psychiatric Safari used this argument to encourage compliance: 'If you had diabetes, you would take insulin, wouldn't you? It's exactly the same thing.' (Except, it's not. Though ironically there is a theory that anti-depressants make you more susceptible to type 2 diabetes because of weight gain.)

Some anti-depressants, such as **amitriptyline** and **trazodone** – given at a low dose – are said to help with insomnia. At the time I was given it, I felt the latter helped me between my first Sleepless Skirmish and my big Insomnia Crash, four years later. But when things got really bad, it was hopeless.

What often happens is that your sleeplessness forms part of a psychiatric diagnosis and one or more types of drug start to be added in.

It's also important to mention that newer studies suggest that anti-depressants come with issues around dependence and withdrawal. For decades, the psychiatric 'establishment' insisted that 'discontinuation syndrome' was 'mild, and self-limiting'. But as this book goes to print, 76 million anti-depressants are being prescribed a year and 17 per cent of the UK population are on them. Many experts believe this is because they're too unpleasant to come off.

22nd July

0 HOURS, 0 MINUTES

My husband has moved to the spare room. The first night, the sleeping pills did not work. Last night, I took two. It didn't make any difference.

23rd July

0 HOURS, 0 MINUTES

I come from a medical family and have always been sceptical about alternative therapies (rightly or wrongly – discuss). One of my favourite health-related books is the 2001 *Snake Oil and Other Preoccupations* by the late journalist John Diamond, described by the *Observer* as a 'fresh and feisty . . . unfinished polemic against the delusions of alternative medicine'. The brilliant Diamond, who was married to food writer Nigella Lawson, died of cancer before he could finish his work.

Even with this cynicism in mind, I am so desperate, I decide to junk my principles and try an alternative therapy that I've heard good things about. Calling around in my lunch hour, I find an acupuncturist who fits me in with an emergency appointment. I spend 40 minutes telling her my medical history and the problems I am currently having. Then I subject myself to the porcupine treatment and hope for instant results.

She is very nice but it doesn't work.

Tomorrow I will move on to the next potential solution.

NOTE: *I know that many therapies (especially alternative ones) are not supposed to work in one 'hit' and you have to give them time. In fact, at some point in the next couple of years, I will try acupuncture again and have a course of several sessions. But right now, I'm in such a state – and my mind is fluttering so wildly all over the place – that I am more impatient than usual (which is saying something) and expect an instant fix.*

24th–26th July

0 HOURS, 0 MINUTES

I race around new-agey Covent Garden in my lunch breaks, looking for solutions. Aromatherapy massage, reiki – I think a purple crystal is even thrown in at some point. 'Woo-woo' shit but I am desperate.

These don't work, either.

27th July

0 HOURS, 0 MINUTES

I am a fit person, proud of my figure, and I try to continue my regime at my Power Plate class, knowing exercise is key to sleep. But my arms can't support my body to do press-ups, my legs buckle. My limbs feel like overcooked spaghetti.

I'm not sure if this is because of the sleeping pills (I've read somewhere that they can impair muscle strength and balance) or I am just so fatigued my body is starting to fail.

29th July

O HOURS, O MINUTES

I visit a hypnotist who works locally out of a damp, smelly room. Admittedly, in my dashing-about desperation, I haven't done my due diligence into the aspect of his 'clinic'. It's close to the main road, there is a noisy, old-fashioned air-conditioning unit and the guy himself looks like Arthur Pewty, a *Monty Python* character played by Michael Palin.

The plasticky chair sticks to my legs in the summer heat.

Arthur's voice is no more prepossessing than his appearance. I try very hard to submit to his trance-inducing charms but it's impossible to count down to total zen with a bus thundering past.

The hypnotist says that maybe I'll have more luck in the comfort of my own home. So he sells me a CD (these are the days before apps) of one of those 'progressive relaxation' exercises where you loosen the muscles in one part of the body after another. The aim is that you'll become so relaxed you eventually fall asleep.

I spend several consecutive nights trying to drop off with a heavy laptop beside me on the bed, listening to the CD. (See note on 'trying', below.)

It doesn't work.

31st July

O HOURS, O MINUTES

'Why don't you just "try" to sleep?' ask friends and family. I'm losing count of the number of times I have heard this. Good advice, arguably, but, if you think about it for a moment, 'trying' is about the worst thing you can do because it implies effort. Surely sleep is about the opposite of trying?

And anyway, how does one 'try' to sleep, exactly? It's not as though I am tossing and turning after an ecstasy-fuelled rave. I'm in bed, it's dark – what else am I supposed to do? Lie rigid under the duvet with my eyes screwed shut? Those relaxation exercises are just not 'doing it' for me in my hyper-alert state.

Surely, as soon as sleep becomes a conscious effort, you are on to a loser.

I know I have sadness around the end of my marriage as well as uncertainty about the future, mixed with a large dollop of fear. But my continued sleeplessness feels dispro-portionate. It's as though my insomnia is morphing into a 'standalone' problem.

NOTE ON 'O HOURS, O MINUTES': *This 'Bridget Jones'-style nihilism about the hours I did not sleep may become boring. And possibly a bit incredible. In fact, in common with my family, friends and doctors, you may not believe it at all. And you know what? I don't blame you for a second.*

But even now, as I write this book, I truly believe I didn't sleep for all those years. And despite consulting many sleep experts, I continue to argue furiously that I never entered snoozy unconsciousness during my Insomnia Crash.

This debate – when a person says they haven't slept but science and common sense insist that surely they have – is known as paradoxical insomnia. I go into it more on page 189.

How much sleep do you really need and when should you get it?

There is received wisdom about how many hours a person 'should' sleep. (And it's a popular subject: a quick Google of 'how much sleep is healthy' yields 612 million results.)

The oft-quoted magic number is eight hours. Some recently-leaked-but-haven't-yet-actually-materialized government guidelines were going to suggest we should sleep between seven and nine hours, so an average of eight. The magic number is bandied about like the holy grail. Fail to 'achieve' it and you have done just that, failed. Which means you are destined for miserable, exhausted days when you trip over kerbs, crave carbohydrates and can't work or socialize properly.

This figure hasn't been pulled out of the air: there have been several studies backing it up. A recent American paper agreed that a minimum of seven hours is recommended for good health. The research was based on hundreds of studies which followed people's long-term experience of heart disease, diabetes and mental health difficulties. Those who slept between seven and nine hours were typically at lower risk of future ill health, hence the recommendation.

This follows a study in the peer-reviewed scientific journal *Sleep*. Almost 1.4 million adults were followed by researchers at Warwick Medical School and the University of Naples medical school. The research found that 6 hours' sleep or less was associated with a 12 per cent increased risk of premature death. Research conducted in a 2019 study had similar results.

The time you need to spend unconscious varies with age. One source detailed that 18–60-year-olds 'need' 7 hours or more, 61–64-year-olds 'need' 7–9, and the over 65s drop an hour again (for some unspecified reason).

'Why seven or eight hours seems to be the magic number is unclear,' said the report's author. 'But don't underestimate the importance of a good night's sleep.' Helpful.

But. And there is a but. Depending on certain variables, including your genetic make-up, age and lifestyle, your 'perfect' amount might fall outside this range.

To my sleep guru, Dr Sophie Bostock, this area of research is familiar. 'Just like your shoe size or height, "optimum sleep" varies from person to person,' she says. 'For example, some people have a "short sleep" gene which means they feel alert and refreshed after just five or six hours' rest.'

Other experts express the view that if you can function on four or five hours a night, can complete tasks and don't feel tired – well, then you are getting enough.

Donald Trump and Margaret Thatcher both famously claimed they needed only four hours' sleep to operate effectively (hmm). Sadly, you can't train yourself to do that. But is it possible to work out your personal magic number, or at least the fewest hours' sleep you can get away with, and still feel OK?

The answer is apparently to go to sleep when you feel tired and wake up without an alarm. Then do the maths. Says

Dr Bostock: 'If you wake up naturally without an alarm, feel refreshed and don't need caffeine, sugar or a nap to get through the day, then you're probably getting enough.'

So perhaps your body decides your own, personal magic number. But 0 hours, 0 minutes is not enough for even the hardiest sleep-warrior.

NOTE: *It is apparently possible to sleep for too long. The Warwick and Naples study also found a 30 per cent rise in risk of death for people who slept 9 hours or more, possibly because they may have underlying medical or social problems. Interestingly, the report concluded that while short sleep may represent a cause of ill health, long sleep is believed to represent an indicator of ill health.*

2nd August

0 HOURS, 0 MINUTES

After two weeks without sleep, I am quivering at my desk. Normally a decisive, confident person, I now stare blankly at my team when they ask for direction. I have to keep working. Havetohaveto. If I lose that, I lose everything. Not only will I require the cash if I'm going to survive as a single mum, I am going to need the self-esteem and validation that comes from having an interesting and (kind of) important job.

But I simply cannot perform. I stare at the page proofs. Half the time, I hide in the loos, fighting off a panic attack. I have never had a panic attack before but I imagine this is one – my heart is racing, my vision has gone blurry and I can't sit still. I can tell my staff feel baffled by and uncomfortable about this change in their boss, though they are too polite to say anything. But they are kind. Cups of tea appear magically on my desk.

At some point this morning, I am sent an email by a TV company, asking me to appear on their morning show to talk about a celebrity who has endorsed breastfeeding.

Normally unfazed by this sort of request, I sit there staring at my computer screen for an hour, unable to decide whether to participate. 'Should I do this?' I ask my new, 23-year-old graduate assistant.

29th August

O HOURS, O MINUTES

Last night I took an overdose of my anti-depressant, trazodone. I didn't want to die. I wanted to sleep and hoped there might be some hazy benefit from emptying the blister pack.

There wasn't.

The world tilted alarmingly and I was violently sick, emptying some of last night's Rioja onto our newish loft extension carpet. Frightened, I called an ambulance. I don't recall a great deal about what happened at hospital, except that I was given an anti-emetic, plugged into a saline drip and made to feel like one of those moronic time-wasters who calls the emergency services when their cat is stuck on a roof.

I get a taxi home (alone) about three hours later. Later that day, my boss – who doesn't know what happened and continues to be sympathetic – tells me I should probably go on sick leave. Take as long as you need, she says. Your job will be here when you are ready to come back.

30th August

0 HOURS, 0 MINUTES

I have taken to ringing friends and family members, asking them for unspecified help they are powerless to provide. (Usually along the lines of: 'I need to sleep, please help me sleep.') For the first couple of conversations, they are patient and sympathetic. But as my friends are usually at work, subsequent pleas become irritating. Eventually, my calls are screened.

My sister-in-law tells me I phoned her 30 times yesterday.

3rd September

0 HOURS, 0 MINUTES

I am helplessly watching my life fall apart, piece by piece. Like one of those dreams, where you are awake but somehow tied down so you can't run.

Or an operation where the anaesthetic hasn't worked properly and you are screaming but the surgeons ignore you.

As if it were all happening to someone else.

8th September

0 HOURS, 0 MINUTES

Back to school. I am terrified. Our small primary school is a close-knit and friendly community, but it's also a hive of gossip. I really don't need this.

I drop my kids at the school gate and aim to dash back to the car as quickly as possible. But – too late – I am faced by several of the Mummy Corps marching their offspring down the street.

My Insomnia Crash happened just as school was breaking up for the summer and I haven't seen any of the gang since early July. Over the summer, the cheerful working mum they saw at book club has become a fidgety ghost, who suddenly finds it difficult to make eye contact.

I know I don't look great but people stop chatting when they see me. One woman actually does a double take, like they do in the movies. I give a falsely bright smile, exchange some 'how was your summer?'s and dash back to the car.

My husband and I have retained a part-time nanny to do 'pick up' – a necessity on those days when I was working in town. In the mornings, we do a rota with another family. More and more, I beg our friends to take the kids into school, even on 'our' days. They are very kind and oblige, though I start to feel guilty for not pulling my weight. Even something as simple as the school run is excruciating now, however much I want to be there for my children.

17th September

0 HOURS, 0 MINUTES

It's now eight weeks since I stopped being able to sleep. I have been referred to a consultant psychiatrist at an NHS hospital. The sleeping tablets and anti-depressants prescribed by my GP haven't worked. The time at home on sick leave has not helped – if anything, I have got worse. I have been spending a lot of the day in bed, trying to sleep or 'reading' (which means gazing at those black, squiggly marks presented in lines on a sheet of paper. I can't actually put them in order and make any sense of them).

Sitting in the consultant's office, I am so exhausted I can hardly say a word.

The softly spoken doctor is sympathetic but, just to make sure, I beg him to prescribe me something that will 'buy' me some rest. I am practically hugging him round the knees. The psychiatrist listens intently to the story of my domestic upheaval and how my distress has plunged me headlong into disabling insomnia.

He agrees that I need a bit of extra help, so 'ups' my anti-depressant and prescribes me a tranquillizer called clonazepam – part of the benzodiazepine drug family, a.k.a. 'benzos'.

So begins my Psychiatric Safari: an eight-year love affair with pills in colourful boxes with seductive names, like Seroquel and Lyrica.

Somewhere in the recesses of my squeezed-lemon brain, I know that clonazepam is part of the same family as diazepam (a.k.a. Valium) and that these drugs have been discredited for a number of conditions for which they used to be widely prescribed. But right now, I couldn't give a damn.

When you are likely to be referred to a psychiatrist and what might happen

In the UK, almost all cases of insomnia are treated by your NHS family doctor. However, this isn't the case for everyone (waves hand from the back of the class).

NB: If you have private medical insurance, or the means to afford a private psychiatrist, you may find yourself in a specialist's office sooner rather than later.

It's important to mention at this point that psychiatry is different from other areas of medicine. There's no question that your consultant will want to help you in your distress. And nothing in medicine is 'black and white'. But for obvious reasons, a field that deals in emotions and the inner workings of your mind has more room for opinions and differing approaches than, say, dermatology.

Some doctors think that drugs are useful, others, less so.

Dr Sami Timimi is a senior consultant child and adolescent psychiatrist and visiting professor of child psychiatry and mental health Improvement. 'Insomnia is very common as a part of the presenting problem in psychiatry,' he says. 'But it's rarely the reason for the referral on the GP's letter. That is generally framed as depression or anxiety.'

According to Dr Timimi, from the minute you walk into a psychiatrist's office, you are being assessed.

'We have the GP's letter in front of us but we also extract phenomenology,' he says. This means that the doctor is listening to what you are saying, how you are saying it and your body language. He or she will be conducting a 'mental status examination', taking into account your appearance and behaviour, at the same time as taking a medical history. 'Your doctor will be working out which category you fit in the ICD (International Classification of Diseases),' says Dr Timimi. 'If you have difficulty falling asleep, psychiatrists will usually relate it to anxiety. If you wake up early, we'll think: depression. The categorization you get is then meant to determine your treatment pathway.'

There are generally three alleyways down which you and your insomnia might gallivant. Here follows some chat about prescription drugs.

The other avenues are 'talking therapies' (see page 60) and, increasingly, digital interventions/apps such as Sleepio (see page 5 and Resources on page 283).

Drugs: More often than not, a psychiatrist will prescribe medication. If you're not already on a psychotropic (psychotropic = affecting a person's mental state) drug, you'll almost certainly be started on something. If you are already taking tablets, the dose will likely be increased or you'll be switched to a different kind of pill, or a new medication will be added.

'Whether you are diagnosed with depression or anxiety, the irony is that the drug treatment is pretty much the same thing,' says Dr Timimi. 'The first line is usually the prescription of an SSRI (a selective serotonin reuptake inhibitor) or an SNRI' (a related class of drug – the 'N' stands for norepinephrine). Both change the concentration of certain chemicals found in the brain and some other parts of the body.

'The theory is that these drugs, usually referred to as "anti-depressants", take two to four weeks to work fully,' says Dr Timimi. 'Everyone's reaction to these drugs is different. It's analogous to alcohol. Some people become sleepy, some happy and others violent.'

Despite the changes in the NICE guidelines, some doctors still prescribe benzodiazepines for insomnia (see page 29). 'Personally, I do not prescribe benzos,' says Dr Timimi. 'Sometimes to help with sleep I prescribe promethazine, which is an antihistamine – it's a similar ingredient to the one that is in Nytol, the over-the-counter sleep aid you can buy at the chemist.

'All pharmacological remedies – however mild – have issues around addiction and withdrawal and can create rebound insomnia. Rebound insomnia is defined as difficulty initiating or maintaining sleep that is worsened in the context of the abrupt discontinuation of sleeping pills.'

Are you starting to see the problem here?

At the end of your appointment, you'll be scheduled in for a follow-up. 'If you aren't seen to be recovering by the next session, many psychiatrists will either increase the medication or add in another drug,' says Dr Timimi.

It's important to mention at this point that certain people *are* helped by psychotropic medication – especially those with more severe 'disorders'. Which, of course, is vital – and, in some cases, literally a lifesaver.

But it's not the same for everyone and many of the more enlightened psychiatrists admit problems with the automatic prescription of tablets. 'From the moment you turn up, you are hitched to a diagnosis,' says Dr Timimi. 'But we rarely tell people that a psychiatric diagnosis doesn't explain anything. To say that someone's low mood is caused by depression is like saying that a pain in the head is caused by a headache. Diagnoses in psychiatry are just short-hand descriptions but they do not explain why you feel or behave the way you do.

'A year down the road, you could find yourself on several medications. As more drugs are added, your brain becomes a "chemical soup".'

Chemical soup. Hmm. I was to find myself drowning in a vat of it.

8th October

0 HOURS, 0 MINUTES

Though I am mentally exhausted and unable to put two sensible words together, I have frantic periods of activity where I race around the country, hoping that a new location might magically bring sleep. (So this is what chickens do when their heads are separated from their bodies. I now identify with those poor, decapitated hens.)

Right now, I'm on a tramline up and down the M1 to my brother and sister-in-law's place in the country. I later realize that it's probably not safe for me to drive but I'm on autopilot, crawling up the inside lane at 60mph. I've already discovered that my parents' home is not soothing. For one, it's no longer my childhood bedroom. It's in a newish house with none of my things in it.

I spend the odd night at the home of several local close friends, thinking there might be a trick/genre of bed I haven't tried that holds the secret. There isn't. I annoy the parents and freak out the kids with my distracted antsy-ness.

None of this works and I'm starting to disturb the sleep of others. One family looks drained and resentful the next morning – apparently I kept them awake by flushing their noisy toilet several times during the night.

At home, I still try different variations. Two pillows, one pillow, no pillow. Someone recommends a spiky purple rubber yoga mat you lie on, on the floor.

Meanwhile, I spend most of the day in or on my bed, inwardly gibbering (at some point I start outwardly gibbering). My eventually-to-be-ex husband and I are in stalemate.

Throughout this whole period, I am lucky that my kids are taken care of by a supportive school that hugs them close, a succession of kind after-school nannies and, of course, my ex.

NOTE: *The situation is desperately sad and will be for years. But this book isn't about my family. At the time of writing, my kids are teenagers and starting to get on with their lives. This is about me and my non-sleep.*

15th November

0 HOURS, 0 MINUTES

After three months 'off sick', I am due to return to work. The problem is, I am no better than when I packed up in August. In fact, I am worse. Maybe I can just 'power through' it? A case of mind over matter? The 'old Miranda' could be pretty determined.

But I feel like shit and am terrified of a) getting on the Tube and b) facing my colleagues again. I put on one of my black, pre-Insomnia Crash, kick-ass editor dresses, a slick of my old go-to bright red lipstick and a pair of heels. I know I look a bit cadaverous. A cream-faced loon.

I pop an extra clonazepam.

My friend N has offered to drive me to the station and even travel down on the Tube with me for moral support. I open the front door to her. She suggests perhaps I might try some more toned-down make-up and maybe a more forgiving dress colour?

N hand-holds me to central London. She bids me fare-well outside the magazine building, though I'd rather like to bring her inside with me, like my mummy on the first day of school. I take a deep breath, head past reception and push the second-floor lift button. Outside the actual office, I feel so weak and so nervous, I think I might actually faint.

But people have either been well-briefed or they are just incredibly tactful: there is no staring or gawping. I am met with a sprig of lavender on my desk and a box of Earl Grey. People act as if I've just come back from a short break (but without the 'did you have a good holiday?' or 'how is your baby doing?').

Mondays on the magazine start with a catch-up meeting, to see how the team is progressing with deadlines, production, photography, etc. I used to preside over these, sitting boss-ishly on the corner of a desk, cheerleading and cajoling. This morning, I just take a seat with the rest of the team.

My second-in-command has been 'acting up' as editor. She skilfully oversees the session while I frown meaningfully at the printed schedule in front of me (for meaningfully, read meaninglessly).

But from this very first meeting, things do not feel right. I am disorientated with exhaustion and possibly a bit woozy from the clonazepam. I can't engage. All I want is to escape to the loos.

My deputy is really good at managing the magazine. She has passion and flair and has absolutely grown into the role in my absence. So, for this month, while I am bedding back in, our roles are to be reversed. I am to take the 'number two' role and do more nitty-gritty copy editing. But tasks I would have previously swooshed through in five minutes take me hours. In fact, I don't complete them. Should a comma go here? This paragraph needs moving but I have no idea where it should go.

Worryingly, I am starting to ask myself: do I really care about baby-led weaning and small motor development anymore?

I note that my friend T has landed the plum job on a sister magazine – the job I was about to apply for before my world took a dive. On one level I am pleased for her; she's a talented journalist. I'm not jealous, exactly, because there is no way I could do that job right now. But it does make my failings seem greater.

Rushing off to the loo again, I give myself a pathetic pep talk in the mirror. On one occasion I (silently) scream at my reflection. I go back to my desk, where I try to act 'normal'. Fifteen minutes later I am back in the bathroom.

My colleagues must think I have a serious bowel problem – or perhaps a cocaine habit.

Somehow I make it to 5.30pm. I can't face the Underground rush hour, so I get a black cab all the way to north London. It costs an absolute fortune.

19th November

O HOURS, O MINUTES

The fourth day of this charade (in fact, the third – I didn't make it in at all on the Wednesday). I sit down with my boss, who looks concerned.

We agree that I should go 'off sick' again.

What makes someone go from temporarily sleepless to a full-blown chronic insomniac?

'It all depends on the "three Ps",' says Dr Sophie Bostock. 'Predisposing, precipitating and perpetuating factors.'

Predisposing factors:

These are characteristics which put you at greater risk but by themselves are not enough to cause insomnia. For example, your genetic predisposition, or being older or female. Or being a worrier.

Precipitating factors:

This is the stuff that 'triggers' you, usually associated with stress of some kind: a new job, family conflict, work problems, changes in schedules (shift work, etc.).

Perpetuating factors:

Crucially, the perpetuating factors affect you not just in terms of disrupted sleep but also in terms of patterns of thinking or behaviour which keep the problem going. (See page 215 on cognitive behavioural therapy for insomnia, CBTi.)

One of these Ps on its own might not result in insomnia – it's the combination that matters. Some people watch TV in bed every night and claim to sleep really well. But they might not have a previous history, a caffeine habit and a stressful occupation.

Year Two

23rd January

32 MINUTES, 5 MINUTES, 1 HOUR, 7 MINUTES

The clonazepam periodically buys me some snatched periods of sleep and a pleasant fuzziness in the hours between. But this relief is haphazard and doesn't last. I need more of the stuff to get the same result, then more again.

At my first follow-up, the consultant increases the prescription. At a later date he ups it again over the phone.

Tonight, I tell myself I'm going to try to stick to the prescribed dose, hiding the extras in one of my boots as an 'emergency stash'. Then the early hours – it's an emergency! – see me rooting around in the dark to avail myself of said stash.

This is not good.

Tossing and Turning

Year Two

15th March

O HOURS, O MINUTES

The thing about sleep is that, like breathing or eating, everyone does it. (Or not, if they have insomnia.) This means that everyone has an opinion based on their 'own experience', which they are not averse to sharing.

The motive behind this is almost invariably well-meaning. It's just that some of the advice – especially if given by eight-hours-a-nighters – can feel frustrating. People can be casually careless and even a bit smug. Some of them, one wants to throttle, especially those who say: 'Oh really, poor you. How terrible that must be. But I've always slept SO well. Head on the pillow, and BANG, nine hours later, it's the morning.'

Some other bits of counsel that have come my way over the last nine months or so:

Try medication. A big subject. Sleeping pills can be helpful in the short term, but they have diminishing returns. And you can get hooked on them. (As we shall see.)

Don't try medication. I totally respect those people who cured their insomnia with Jo Malone lavender and lovage candles and camomile tea. It doesn't appear to work for me.

Eat more carbs, eat fewer carbs. One study found that post-menopausal women who consumed a diet high in refined carbohydrates – particularly sugar – were more likely to develop insomnia. Whereas another paper insisted that, when eaten four hours before bedtime, carbs may boost tryptophan and serotonin (see below).

Eat foods containing tryptophan. This is an amino acid that apparently turns into the feel-good hormone serotonin. It's said to convert into the hormone melatonin, which promotes sleep. You can find tryptophan in turkey, nuts and seeds, kidney beans and turnips. Didn't work for me and made me feel a bit unwell.

Get a sleep tracker which will prove you do sleep, actually. Except one night, my tracker told me I was sleeping when I was down in the kitchen making some toast. (See page 161 for more on bloody sleep trackers.)

Try cognitive behavioural therapy (CBT). The NHS website defines CBT as 'a talking therapy that can help you manage your problems by changing the way you think, and your behavioural strategies'. Sounds great but right now I am too flattened by exhaustion to even understand the phrase 'behavioural strategy'. 'Plain' CBT is actually quite different from CBTi (the 'i' stands for insomnia), the specialized and more super version. (See page 215.)

Other suggestions include: Put lavender oil on your pillow; spray magnesium on your arm (suspiciously white and gloopy); try biofeedback (some weird monitoring of your vital signs); stop taking naps (haven't taken a nap since I was three).

Give up coffee. Give that person an NVQ.

I stick with the clonazepam.

Year Ten: A note from the future

SPOILER ALERT! You've probably sussed that – for this book to have been written in the first place – I made some sort of recovery.

At this point in my Insomnia Crash narrative, however, things got a bit wobbly.

Please indulge me if I don't have an entry for every week or even every month; I was certainly incapable of keeping a traditional journal at the time. In the entry for 19th March (nine months or so into my ordeal) and for the next few years, I remembered and recorded impressions, vignettes, snatches of conversations and faces. There are gaps simply because every day was generally the same as the last and really too boring to write about, let alone read.

Yet in another sense – an emotional one, perhaps – I remember everything.

Even now, things are coming back to me, often at the strangest moments: when I'm in the bath, say, or driving. Many of these memories are painful. I am also shocked by the thoughts (if that's what you can call the repetitive meanderings) that went through my head back then. The things I was saying or doing; my lack of insight and logic.

And most of all, my complete sense of humour failure.

To argue that I wasn't responsible for my thoughts, words or actions is trite and a bit of a cop-out. But it's very difficult to think, talk and do when you haven't slept for months.

Which, when enough of the months are laid end-to-end, turn into years.

Some of the material to come may be quite upsetting for those who have, or may have had, mental health problems (not necessarily related to insomnia) or thoughts of self-harm.

19th March

0 HOURS, 0 MINUTES

I find myself wondering if you can die from insomnia. I do some research. There *is* a super-rare but fatal condition called fatal familiar insomnia (FFI) and I'm sure I have it.

Before you start Googling too, it's *very* unlikely that you have FFI. It's a genetic mutation, a bit like CJD (linked to mad cow disease), which has only affected a handful of families, mainly in Germany and Italy.

7th April

O HOURS, O MINUTES

The radio keeps me up to date with certain events. Indeed, my Insomnia Crash has two newsy bookends: the story of the Chilean miners stuck far underground and those Thai schoolboys marooned in Tham Luang cave, eventually to be rescued by divers. These reports speak to me a) because they feature a terrifyingly claustrophobic setting (I am terribly claustrophobic) and b) I kind of identify with them.

Yes, I spend my days on a comfortable mattress in a spacious loft conversion with natural light and a book, not in a sunless tunnel. There is food in the kitchen downstairs; I am not dependent on tin cans dropped down a mine shaft. I could leave the house at any moment I want and go anywhere in the world.

But I can't read because my concentration is shot. I only go downstairs when I really have to. More often than not, I make toast and bring it upstairs. (I am to eat a lot of toast in the sleepless years.) And at some point in year three, I stop leaving the house altogether.

So what kept the Chilean miners and Thai schoolboys going? Or, further back, guys like Terry Waite, the Archbishop's envoy chained to a Lebanese radiator from 1987 to 1991? Or anyone with some sort of long-term prison sentence, whether it has been bestowed by a judge or by unfortunate circumstance?

The answer, I'm finding, is that you simply have no choice.

Night falls, day arrives and still you are there.

And each morning, you hope against hope that the day will be better, even if there's no evidence that it will be. That's optimism. Maybe that's what it is to be human.

5th June

O HOURS, O MINUTES

Every day is the same, yet tougher than the last, in a sort of super-dystopian *Groundhog Day*.

Will this 24-hour circuit never stop? Even Le Mans is only for one day. Sticking with the racing-car analogy, life is a bit like being forever in the groove of my brother's 1970s Scalextric track. Though at least even that juddered to a halt some of the time. (Most of the time, in fact.)

Evidence suggests that my temporary 'off button' has had a fatal malfunction. So maybe the only way to end this horror is to switch myself off, permanently. The idea of suicide pops into my head. Then it stays.

My obsessive help-seeking behaviour moves to the laptop. I Google: suicide, best way. Then: suicide, painless; suicide, peaceful. I am not happy with the solutions (they look painful, messy and not at all peaceful).

This is when the websites start to appear.

Obviously, I am not going to name them. In fact, investigating now, from some years in the future, many of them appear to have been taken down. This is a good thing. Not only were they full of 'methods' and suggestions (yep), they also had places to leave messages and hook up with others who want to 'catch the bus' with you.

Yes, 'catch the bus'. What a homely metaphor to describe leaving the earth in a violent way, destroying the lives of everyone you hold dear.

I learn some important information. Never overdose on paracetamol, people, if you want to avoid a lingering, painful death four days after you have changed your mind and decided you want to live after all. Your liver is already screwed beyond repair.

For a while, I become obsessed with obtaining Nembutal, the drug on which Marilyn Monroe glamorously overdosed in 1962. Nembutal is an old-fashioned tranquillizer called a barbiturate, rare as a unicorn. I read they use Nembutal in the Dignitas assisted suicide clinic in Switzerland (bookmarked for another day's Googling), which is for people in the terminal stages of dreadful illnesses such as motor neurone disease.

In my deranged state, I think that if I keep Googling and Googling the very same phrase, hundreds of times a day, a different solution will appear.

Of course, I do not really want to die. But I want to get off this eternal treadmill. I want to sleep.

6th June

0 HOURS, 0 MINUTES

I am very interested in Dignitas and spend several hours on the website. I download the application forms.

You may be surprised to hear it's quite difficult to get into an assisted suicide clinic.

What to do if you feel suicidal

The following information has been adapted from the MIND website (see Resources on page 283).

What does it mean to feel 'suicidal'?

Many people think about suicide at some point in their life. It's a lonely, overwhelming and terrifying place to be.

The tragedy is that 800,000 people worldwide do take their lives every year (7,000 in the UK). The majority are young men. Women are more likely to 'attempt' suicide and not succeed. One reason given for this disparity is that men use more violent means.

Imagine, then, how many people must toy fleetingly with the idea of taking their own lives.

Suicidal feelings come in many forms. Some people have abstract thoughts that they 'can't go on', that ending their lives might be preferable to the current hell. Or that family and friends would be better off without them.

These feelings may come on suddenly, build over time or might change from moment to moment.

If you are thinking about ways of killing yourself, or starting to make plans, seek help right NOW.

If you are feeling suicidal:

- If thoughts around suicide are all-consuming and you actually think you might hurt yourself, go straight to hospital or call the emergency services and ask for an ambulance.

- Tell someone. If you can't or don't want to speak to a family member or friend, call your doctor.
- If you don't have this option, or don't want to speak to someone you know, there are various organizations and charities that can provide support. See Resources on page 283.

A suicidal person might feel:
- hopeless and desperate, like there is no point in living
- tearful and overwhelmed by negative thoughts
- in unbearable pain that they can't imagine ending
- useless, like everyone would be better off without them
- cut off from their body or physically numb
- fascinated by death

They might experience:
- poor sleep, particularly early waking (if, indeed, they sleep at all)
- eating less and losing weight, or the opposite
- lack of interest in their physical appearance, so that it's neglected
- wanting to avoid others
- making a will or giving away possessions
- self-loathing and low self-esteem
- urges to harm themselves

Suicidal thoughts are not permanent.

They are just that, thoughts. Things have a tendency to get better, even if those in pain can't see it right now.

But suicidal actions can be permanent.

NOTE: *After I 'got better', I discovered this, from the Austrian poet, Rainer Maria Rilke:*

> *Let everything happen to you*
> *Beauty and terror*
> *Just keep going*
> *No feeling is final.*

I wish I had known this poem during my Insomnia Crash. Although, more likely than not, I would have told it to fuck off.

I'm certain I wouldn't have been able to process its wise message but, from this lofty, comfortable place of hindsight, I think it's wonderful. It helps me on normal 'bad days' and I have stuck it above my desk.

Maybe it will help me if I find myself here again.

17th June

0 HOURS, 0 MINUTES

How I spend the days

Demarcating what constitutes a 'day' is tricky when you don't have a 'night' to split up the 24 (48, 72, 96, etc.) hour time unit. The pattern varies a bit but I normally give up the ghost around 3.30am and go downstairs to make some toast. I know I should wait longer but I'm *hungry*. Apparently, there are medical reasons for my appetite (see page 82). It's not just boredom or gluttony. At least, that's my story.

If the radio hasn't already been on I'll switch it to talkSPORT because I hate music right now – too many difficult emotional associations. Listening to news reminds me of the professional world I have left behind. Sport is good because it's anodyne and not 'triggering'.

At around 6am, I heave a heavy sigh and bring my second breakfast upstairs – normally Weetabix. I try to kid myself that I'm having a jolly breakfast-in-bed treat.

For the first couple of years, I just about manage the school run (sometimes). Thereafter, I wave everyone off for the day and scuttle back upstairs.

I have a bath. Throughout this whole hell, I never miss my bath. I usually have two a day. My baths are, in fact, my sole pleasure. Washing my hair, on the other hand, is trickier because it involves lifting up my arms, which takes energy.

Even if I were to feel like getting properly dressed, there isn't much to choose from because almost all my clothes are magazine-editor, designery, dry clean only and now ridiculously inappropriate. My jeans become first too large as I lose weight, then, later on, too small as I gain it. Besides, denim feels too rough a fabric for days in bed or under a duvet on the sofa. So, it's leggings and T-shirts, pyjamas and, when mine get too small, my ex's pyjamas.

I spend the best part of a decade in or on my bed. Awake.

Most of the time I am mindlessly Googling away: benzodiazepines, suicide or about ideas for a new career (yes, I'm aware of the contradictions here). I decide I might quite like a 'proper' physical illness, a) so someone will look after me and b) because it will be easier for people to understand an *actual* patient and offer sympathy.

If I'm not on the laptop, I'm staring at a book or listening mindlessly to talkSPORT. Sometimes I lug a duvet down to the living room to vacantly watch daytime TV. I try to kid myself I am legitimately 'off sick' – I don't feel my current plight counts, somehow – and attempt to create the cosy, self-indulgent feeling of being home from work with a cold.

This doublethink doesn't work. I am stressed, tense and feel guilty all day long.

(On daytime TV: occasionally a spark of interest breaks through the torpor. I do become fond of a BBC show called *Money for Nothing*, where a perky lady accosts people at the recycling tip, takes their old furniture, adds tassels to it, sells it on for a profit, shows up 'unannounced' at their house and hands over the profit in crisp notes.)

When it's my turn, I pick up the kids from school at around 4pm. In the car on the way home, my conversation is repetitive and annoying. In fact, it's not conversation at all – just a series of rapid-fire questions and non-sequiturs.

For dinner, I rustle up something simple and uninspired that doesn't require thought or coordination. Then I retreat upstairs again as soon as possible. Fire up the laptop. Have another bath.

'Bedtime' is normally around 8.30pm.

Yes, I *know* it's too early. I *know* I should have exercised. I *know* my 'sleep hygiene' has gone to shit. I *know* I shouldn't be staring at a screen all day.

But the next six years pretty much follow this pattern. Tomorrow, and tomorrow, and tomorrow.

How I spend the nights

So, bedtime is the greatest hope time. You never know, *this* could be the night.

I take my pills, lie down optimistically and wait for sleep to creep up on me. I hear the rest of the house go to bed. When I'm still awake an hour later, I'll put on the radio, maybe embark on some obsessive empty-headed web surfing.

Around midnight, I will 'try' to drop off again – but it's hopeless. I have a mental Rolodex spinning around: guilt, regret, fear, random thoughts and an entire lifetime of memories coming back to me. But my wakefulness is due to more than just anxious thoughts. It feels as though I have somehow mislaid the drowsy chemical, that I am physiologically no longer able to shut down.

Morpheus has stopped sprinkling his poppy seeds on my brain; the Sandman has blown away.

By 2am, I'm in despair. Summer nights are the worst. Those early dawns signify failure and make me want to commit mass murder.

I conceive a weird hatred of the part of the year that follows 21st December because it means the days are starting to get lighter again.

1st July

0 HOURS, 0 MINUTES

It amazes me how much sleep enters the lexicon of every-day life. People 'wake up and decide' to do things. They 'sleepwalk their way' through presentations. 'I wouldn't *dream* of doing that,' says a friend.

Every time I hear these phrases (and even find myself saying them), I roll my eyes, bitterly.

12th July

0 HOURS, 0 MINUTES

this sentence doesn't have any punctuation because time
no longer has punctuation not the full stops of night time
and the new sentence of the morning I CAN'T STAND IT
I CAN'T STAND IT HOW AM I EVEN STILL ALIVE

(Apologies to James Joyce.)

13th July

7 HOURS OR SO

Today I *will* sleep and damn the consequences! A devil
overtakes me and I finish the box of clonazepam. While I
actually feel quite pleasant and have read somewhere that
this amount of benzos probably won't do me any harm, I
think that I probably shouldn't have done it and call 999.

Two enormous paramedics turn up, wearing big boots.

On the ambulance ride, I start to feel guilty about my
stupidity and recklessness. Maybe we should turn back?
The paramedics are kind but they're sorry, it doesn't work
like that. They reassure me that calling them was the right
thing to do; it's best to be safe. 'We'll help you get the help
you need,' they say.

The A&E nurses, on the other hand, are not kind. They
are perfunctory, silent and unsmiling when taking my
blood pressure and temperature. I don't even get any pre-
cautionary saline this time.

I am led to a plastic side room with blue plastic seats
that are impossible to sit on: they are slopey, the 'bum area'

is too small and I keep sliding off. The chairs are festooned with round cigarette burns. Five hours, I sit there. I try to see the upside: there are some new walls to stare at for a while.

As I regard the walls, I'm trying to work out exactly why I have taken all these pills. Is it that old cliché, a 'cry for help'? The thing is, I *have* cried out for help. I cry out for help every day. The medical professionals know I'm here. But the only help there seems to be is drugs. More and more of them, all the time. Which is seeming less and less like a good idea. (And they don't get me any sleep.)

Finally, a youngish mental health nurse appears. We have a brief chat where I spin out the same old complaints and I am referred to something called the Home Treatment Team, whose job it is to keep people out of psychiatric hospitals.

The Home Treatment Team say they will pay me a visit tomorrow.

A happy coda to a grim day: when I get home, the clonazepam still in my system sends me to sleep for seven hours.

My joy cannot be overstated. This is clearly not a workable strategy but the next morning I open my eyes in astonishment and delight at having finally had some rest.

16th July

1 HOUR, 15 MINUTES (SMALL CLONAZEPAM HANGOVER)

I'm not entirely impressed with the Home Treatment Team, who are to pop up at various junctures in the next few years of my Insomnia Crash. For a start, you rarely see the same person twice. There is no 'treatment' or therapy. The Home Treaters arrive in the early evening, ask how you are doing, but don't really listen to the response.

Given all I say every night is, 'I didn't sleep again . . . I can't sleep . . . I can't sleep,' it must be quite boring for them.

Each Treater takes their shoes off, sits down on an armchair and noisily flips open a heavy, black, old-fashioned briefcase (they all seem to have the same one: do they share it?) to give you your pills, which – rightly, in this case – they don't trust you to dispense yourself. This done, they fill in an illegible medication form.

Then they get the hell out of Dodge and off to their next loony.

5th August

0 HOURS, 0 MINUTES

My boss schedules a meeting in town. I've been off work for a year now (despite that one abortive attempt to return) and something needs to shift.

Knowing my fear of getting on the Tube, my friend A agrees to drive me to town. She helps me choose one of last summer's dresses and some light make-up. I'm nervous about this appointment but my manager couldn't be nicer. The company wants me back, she says. They value me. But maybe I'm not up to editing a magazine right now (you don't say), so why don't I kick-start myself in a more junior capacity? She offers me a job as a features writer on a sister health title, with a view to eventually working back up to my previous level.

This is a great plan in theory. But the truth is I barely remember the alphabet, let alone have the capacity to write meaningful articles offering advice about diet and fitness.

The irony of the subject matter does not escape me.

Friends and family are thrilled for me and say I have to grab the opportunity with both hands. I offer a limp grip.

15th August

0 HOURS, 0 MINUTES

It takes me about two hours to leave the house. I am so jittery, I can't even keep still enough to choose an outfit. I call the editor to say I'm going to be late and it's after 11am by the time I make it into work. I can't face the ten-minute walk to the station, so I drive.

From the first moment I step into the office, everything feels *wrong*.

For starters, the health magazine is on the same open-plan floor as my old parenting title – I can see my former staff beavering away. Then there is the slightly weird situation that this new magazine is the one I was hoping to edit before my Insomnia Crash knocked that one on the head. My friend T, the new editor, is now my boss.

I'm aware that this sounds whiny. And while I'm grateful for the opportunity, Lord Sugar, it's not psychologically the best place to be.

As it happens, I have no legs to stand on, morally. I am hopeless. I am given simple copy to edit but because I no longer have any critical faculty, I tell the editor 'it's fine' and ready for publication. It isn't.

I'm given small pieces to write, real entry-level stuff. I'm not much cop at that, either. It also has to be said I am not best placed to advise on exercise, healthy eating, *sleep*, etc., when I am doing none of the above.

(All this while fielding calls from the Home Treatment Team – the situation could not be more incongruous – alongside dashing in and out of the loo to compose myself.)

The subject matter of the job is not helpful for my new obsession with my physical health. Nor is the extra-fast broadband. While I should be working on editing features, I am Googling 'gum recession'.

Even though I childishly shut down the pages as they walk behind me, I think my colleagues know what is going on.

16th–29th August

0 HOURS, 0 MINUTES

Everyone on the magazine is patient. But after two weeks or so, it's clear the charitable 'back-to-work' scheme is not working on any level.

I arrive (unforgivably) late every day and leave early. Even while my body is sitting on a chair in front of a Mac, I am a useless blob with a fidgety mind. The staff are open-minded journalists who understand mental health issues – but this is not a day-care centre, it's a business.

At some point, my editor friend and I decide it might be better if I work from home. But even then, I turn in half-finished articles and work that would have previously embarrassed me – and would have earned dim looks from me if they had come from one of my team.

I don't recall exactly how it happens but by early September, I am back on sick leave again.

5th September

O HOURS, O MINUTES

I used to have a lot of friends. My best ones let me know they're always there for me. But the more peripheral people have started to melt away. For some of them, it's simply because I'm not 'around' – for drinks after work, coffee after the school run, etc.

Casual acquaintances don't quite know to handle me these days and keep their distance. That's fine with me – I am a small-talk vacuum and very, very boring.

My two closest friends are busy with careers and young families but they still call and come round when they can. I am grateful to them for 'hanging in there' with me, although I can see that they leave visibly upset. We all tend to feel worse after their visits.

When H says she will 'come and sit with me for an hour' – as if I'm an elderly aunt in an old people's home – I know I am done for.

Others offer practical kindnesses. L 'takes' me for walks – like a dog! – in the local woodland; my neighbour K allows me to sit at her table and ramble on circuitously for hours and hours.

There is only ever one subject: me and my health. I have lost the ability to listen to other people, empathize and realize that they might be going through shit in their own lives.

Another L (a beauty journalist) takes me to have free Botox and fillers because it might make me look less frowny and hence feel more cheerful. 'Do I look more like Miranda?' I ask her afterwards. She considers me for a moment. 'Half a Miranda.'

It doesn't work.

5th October

O HOURS, O MINUTES

For most people, sleep is a utility, a kind of 'air bridge' that gets them from one period of activity to the next. But for me, the process of not doing it has become all-consuming.

It's not so much that I feel anxious about the night to come and dread going to bed – though this is common in people with insomnia. It's more that the effects of not sleeping stamp on every daylight hour. I can no longer think creatively, act spontaneously (or act at all, really), feel anything deeply or care about much.

It's what a piece of garlic must feel like: crushed, with a kitchen pestle and mortar. Flattened but also traumatized. Floppy, useless and looking nothing like its original form. And a bit smelly.

This is no way to live.

Year Three

15th January

O HOURS, O MINUTES

The inevitable happens. I receive a letter from my company offering me a redundancy settlement and my P45.

I don't feel mistreated or resentful; they did their best for me and hung in there longer than most other employers would.

I wouldn't go so far as to say it is a good feeling, though.

23rd March

O HOURS, O MINUTES

I am no longer looking outwards, so I turn inwards. My latest obsession is my physical health: specifically, that I am decaying.

Sitting on a bed all day has not been good for my muscle tone. My arms and legs are like sticks, even my feet look skinnier. I keep staring at them. I tell people that my feet are shrinking. They tell me I am insane.

My hair is like straw. I start to see that my white teeth are a little discoloured and the corners of my mouth have begun to turn downwards.

(Even after recovery, I feel there is some truth in all these points. Some of the drugs I was on do cause problems with tooth decay, for example. But at the time, my family tell me it's rubbish, that I am mad, to please shut up. My beleaguered father, a dentist, keeps saying: 'It's mental, not dental.')

At some point in the next few years, I will 'have' pre-cancerous bowel problems (I go for a colonoscopy, where I get extra intravenous benzos, hurray!), osteoporosis (I pay for a private bone-density scan), a too-fast pulse and hormonal problems (I splash out on private Harley Street doctors for the last two).

My results come back normal.

Insomnia: how it affects your physical health

Sleeplessness *does* affect your body.

When people talk about insomnia, they usually refer to it as the symptom of a mental health condition. There's lots of chat about anxiety and depression, and so on. But rarely dwelt on are the physical effects of sleeplessness.

Medical research – and my own personal experiences – bears out that the physical effects of even a short bout of insomnia can be significant and debilitating.

Insomnia is, in fact, linked to a wide variety of conditions, from obesity to type 2 diabetes and even Alzheimer's. The reasons were discussed in the May 2019 edition of the journal *Experimental Psychology*, with theories ranging from blood vessels littered with fatty deposits to 'cellular garbage' in the brain. According to the research, people who sleep less than seven hours a night have a significantly raised level of molecules called microRNAs, which suppress the protein content of cells and have previously been linked to inflammation and poor blood vessel health.

Fantastic.

Partial sleep deprivation . . .

. . . is not as bad as the chronic type. This is when you get some sleep but not as much as you need. Experts refer to this as having a 'sleep debt'.

After one night, you'll feel tired but can normally power through the next day's activities. Following two or three sleepless ones, you'll start to feel exhausted and irritable. Your work performance might be affected, alongside headaches, slowed reactions, memory problems and sluggishness. It's probably dangerous to drive.

Long-term partial sleep deprivation – while not as devastating as total insomnia – is still pretty serious. It's also becoming more common as people use social media, online shopping and 24/7 streaming services.

In one study, researchers followed a group of volunteers who were only allowed to sleep four hours a night for six days on the trot. They developed higher blood pressure, higher levels of the stress hormone cortisol and fewer antibodies in response to a flu vaccine. In a nod to long-term problems, they showed signs of insulin resistance, a precursor to type 2 diabetes.

The good news is that the volunteers' health returned to normal after they made up their sleep debt. But many adults with frantic working lives never quite manage to do this, so it's a cautionary tale.

Chronic insomnia

Clearly, it would be inhumane for scientists to carry out a sleep-deprivation study on a group of people for several years. But researchers have some idea of the devastation inflicted by years of insomnia.

Here, in no particular order, are some of the ways in which sustained sleeplessness can wreak havoc on your body.

Weight gain

The science: Not getting enough sleep makes you more likely to gain weight, according to the analysis of 36 studies, discussed in the journal *Obesity*. (Can you imagine working on the journal *Obesity*? Might stall conversations at parties. Or start them.) Insomnia disrupts the production of ghrelin and leptin – the hormones that control hunger. Thus you crave fatty, starchy and sugary foods, potentially eating hundreds of extra calories a day in refined carbohydrates.

The daytime exhaustion means you can't be bothered to exercise and so your weight spirals – as does a cascade into other conditions such as diabetes and heart disease, discussed below.

What happened to me: For the first six years of my Insomnia Crash, I would say I actually *lost* weight – via muscle tone and even bone density – though an initial test for the latter came back normal. Then, the numbers on the scales started to go up.

For me, this was largely because I was eventually prescribed a drug called olanzapine (see page 145). It's actually an anti-psychotic, a pill primarily used to manage psychosis – a set of symptoms which includes delusions, hallucinations and paranoia, common in those suffering schizophrenia and bipolar disorder. Olanzapine can also be used to 'augment' anti-depressants.

Guess the main side effect of olanzapine?

On top of my chemically-induced ballooning, I was exhausted and miserable, my healthy eating principles long gone. A phobia about leaving the house didn't help in the exercise stakes.

So, I got fat. As this book goes to press, I've been working (with some success) to shift those excess pounds.

Diabetes

The science: A report in the journal *Diabetes Care* found a significant increase in type 2 diabetes in people with chronic insomnia.

Patients who suffered poor sleep (less than five hours a night) for a year or longer had three times the risk of those who slept six hours or more. As with obesity (also linked to type 2 diabetes), the underlying cause is thought to involve disruption of the body's normal hormonal regulation, but in this case it results from insufficient sleep.

What happened to me: At a couple of medical appointments, I was told my sugar levels were raised (the word 'diabetes' was never used and I was never given any medication).

It was obvious I needed to modify my diet, however, and I always got there with a promise to do so before the nurse had a chance to mention it.

My blood sugar is now within the normal range.

Heart disease

The science: In 2019, a top American university published a comprehensive report linking insomnia with high blood pressure.

People who don't get enough sleep also have raised levels of stress hormones and substances that indicate inflammation, a key cause of cardiovascular disease. And the kicker: less than four hours' sleep a night could double a woman's risk of dying of heart disease.

What happened to me: My cholesterol shot up to a moderately serious level. Since I started losing weight, it's better, but still raised. My blood pressure has always been fine.

Dementia/Alzheimer's

The science: Current research indicates that insomnia raises the risk of Alzheimer's. A Harvard Medical School report reckoned that people with sleep problems are nearly 1.7 times as likely to develop cognitive impairments than those without.

One scientific study was particularly terrifying. The author claimed there was 'preliminary evidence' that missing even a single night's sleep could increase levels of a brain protein implicated in Alzheimer's disease.

What happened to me: Pardon? What? Did you say something? My memory isn't what it used to be. So Alzheimer's is in the post. Can this really be right?

Viral infections

The science: It's well known that sleep is necessary for a healthy immune system – the part of our make-up which tackles antigens, or foreign invaders, as well as 'T cells': white blood cells which destroy virus-carrying cells.

A study in the *Archives of Internal Medicine* showed that subjects who slept less than seven hours a night were three times as likely to catch colds than those who got the full eight, or more. Another study found a greater risk of COVID-19 in those who had disrupted sleep, with every one-hour increase in the time spent asleep at night associated with 12 per cent lower odds of catching the virus.

What happened to me: Fortunately, my Insomnia Crash was pre-COVID-19. I don't recall getting particularly more colds – or even a single bout of flu – but this was probably because I didn't leave the house that much and meet that many germs.

Other issues that happened to me

A blood test in year eight threw up some deficiencies in iron, calcium and vitamin D. But iron tablets made me feel sick. A GP buddy advised me that a diet with more red meat and spinach would be sufficient.

The calcium/vitamin D tablets I was prescribed were like eating chalk. So my doctor friend told me that 1000 iu vitamin D3 would suffice. I take vitamin D every day now and do feel better, in an indefinable way.

So are all insomniacs doomed?

The problem is the lack of long-term studies following the same group of people. 'All these chronic conditions are multifactorial, so we need loads of subjects to rule out the impact of confounding factors,' says my sleep guru, Dr Sophie Bostock. 'In the short-term studies, typically healthy people recover after several days of proper sleep.

'We do, however, need projects where we analyse the long-term impacts of improving sleep for insomnia sufferers. The good news is that this is starting to happen because of digital interventions such as apps and online tools which are inherently scaleable.'

And finally, maybe some good news for those of us who have children. 'Parents have been coping with sleep loss for generations,' says Dr Bostock. 'There is no evidence that parents live a shorter time than those who don't have children. In fact, if anything, it's the opposite.'

15th April

O HOURS, O MINUTES

It is not-so-slowly dawning on me that drugs are not the answer to my plight.

I had considered therapy earlier in my Insomnia Crash but didn't think my mind would sit still enough to benefit. It also seemed so American. And self-indulgent. And expensive. But now, this far into my Psychiatric Safari, I feel ready to try. A mutual friend recommends a therapist called Anthony Stone.

Anthony is a gentle septuagenarian giant who lives in north-west London, where therapists outnumber those in need of psychological help. His MO is humanistic psycho-therapy, which Google tells me is: 'the therapeutic model based on humanistic psychology. It is client-centred and recognizes the relationship between therapist and client as significant in creating conditions for growth.'

I'm not really sure what this means but, over the years, Anthony will try a variety of methods to get me 'better'. These include inviting me to hit a cushion with a stick to release assumed anger over elements of my childhood (I don't feel angry and, even if I did, I'm too tired to show it), and examination of the past to try to explain what psycho-logical traumas may have brought me here.

I guess in theory this approach may be helpful to someone who has the capacity for insight. But the problem is that I do not. I am a shell of a person who has not slept for several years. I'm not really in a position to look back and analyse. All I want is to sleep; a dissection of my child-hood can wait.

There are unintended consequences, however. This introspection gives me a new set of disorders to Google.

More than anything, Anthony is disturbed by the amount of pills I am taking. He thinks they have zonked me, made me 'unavailable' and are creating more problems than they solve. As time goes on, he will support my every attempt to get off them, even coming with me to see the original psychiatrist to explain his concerns.

Though the devastation wrought by my sleeplessness is beyond his considerable powers and decades of experience, Anthony sticks by me for years. He can see the person I used to be and does his very best to remind me of her, that she is 'still in there'. He treats me at half price when I stop earning money, sometimes at 30 minutes' notice when I'm feeling particularly desperate. Occasionally, I don't show up at all and Anthony never fails to be understanding.

Anthony arranges to meet me for cups of tea and walks on Hampstead Heath (during the early days, at least, when I am still able to go out). He even comes to visit me in hospital.

Once, when my family go on holiday and I have eaten all the food that is in the house, Anthony brings a parcel of hummus, bread, tomatoes, fruit and chocolate and leaves it at the front door for me.

13th July

O HOURS, O MINUTES

Returning to my room after another fruitless trip to Anthony, I tell myself, 'I give up.' I do this quite frequently:

'Oh, I give up, you've won.' Thing is, I am not entirely sure who the 'you' is. God? Nature? The universe?

But as cheerful Gloucester lamented in King Lear (not surprising he was upset, he'd just had his eyes poked out): 'As flies to wanton boys are we to the gods/They kill us for their sport.'

As in, nothing, or no one, ultimately gives a shit.

And what does 'giving up' mean, anyway? I'm past that actively suicidal bit. You can't give up. You just carry on breathing, feeling worse by the day, while the world rolls on its merry business without you.

Year Four

Nobody in the NHS knows what to do with me.

My local health trust refers me to something called the Complex Care Team. When first they signed me up, it was called the Complex Needs Team. Maybe someone, somewhere, decided that sounded too demanding, wheedly and not very politically correct.

Says the NHS website: 'We provide treatment and support to people with complex mental health problems on the Care Programme Approach (CPA) who do not have a diagnosis of psychosis (schizophrenia, bipolar disorder, psychotic depression and other psychiatric disorders).'

In some ways, it feels quite nice to be 'complex', though I don't like the sound of having 'needs' or being someone who benefits from 'care'. I soon discover that this category is code for people whom the usual psychiatric services have failed to help: in other words, it's a bit of a basket case pick 'n' mix.

Obviously, this *doesn't* really feel nice. It's not so long since I was a financially independent, competent working mother with a wide circle of friends. I could discuss a range of subjects from Shakespeare's late plays to *Sex and the City*. I was able to adapt myself to an audience, ranging from hundreds of industry executives to telling my son's reception class about my job. I wasn't always only able to whine 'I can't sleep' on repeat in front of a mental health worker. My only 'needs' were to have a selection of designer shoes and a foreign holiday from time to time.

Then it gets even worse. I discover that a new and disturbing diagnosis has been slapped on me: Emotionally Unstable Personality Disorder, or EUPD.

Funnily enough, I look it up. According to the *Diagnostic and Statistical Manual*, the *DSM–V*, EUPD (or, to use its old name, Borderline Personality Disorder) is diagnosed on the basis of:

1. a pervasive pattern of instability of interpersonal relationships, self-image and affects, and
2. marked impulsivity beginning by early adulthood and present in a variety of contexts, as indicated by at least five of the following.

Then follows a list that includes 'frantic attempts to avoid real or imagined abandonment'; a pattern of unstable and intense relationships; an unstable 'sense of self'; impulsivity leading to substance abuse and 'reckless driving'; recurrent suicidal behaviour or self-mutilating behaviour; inappropriate intense anger and 'stress-related paranoid ideation'.

Blimey.

I don't really identify with too much of this. My driving is pretty good.

But seriously. The diagnosis really upsets me.

I know I am not an 'easy customer' in the psychiatry supermarket. I am querulous. My conversation (if you can call it that) is repetitive and I don't respond well to advice that to me sounds obvious. I am not recovering as satisfactorily as some other mental health patients. In fact, I am getting worse.

But there was a concrete trigger to my current problems. They did not 'begin in early adulthood'. I was 42.

Three years ago, I had a big life shock, which would have shaken the most stoic of individuals. My response to this trauma – and to me it was a trauma – was to stop sleeping. Everyone responds to trauma in their own way and many, I'm sure, have emotional issues after the end of an important relationship. Protracted insomnia appears to be mine.

I accepted the clinical diagnosis of depression – even if it didn't entirely make sense because my 'illness' came on so suddenly. Anyway, who wouldn't get depressed after years of insomnia, having lost most of the things they had spent their life working for? I didn't particularly see the diagnosis of depression as a value judgement.

An Emotionally Unstable Personality, however?

S, my GP sister-in-law, who has known me for 25 years, does not agree with this diagnosis. But she says it's possible my recent history of half-hearted overdoses counts against me. (A history of 'self-harm' being among the criteria for an EUPD diagnosis, which I thought referred to that sad decision that some young people take to hurt themselves when emotionally distressed.)

Even in my most devastated moments, the thought of taking a razor to my skin is anathema.

And if my benzo 'addiction' is part of the diagnosis, I am hopping with fury.

Who the hell gave me these bloody drugs in the first place? Many EUPD patients have addiction issues. But I've never had a problem with other substances. Despite the odd spot of the usual university binge-drinking. Recreational drugs never really appealed.

S describes patients of hers who have had a diagnosis of EUPD. She assures me that people with this condition generally do not end up top of their year at school, get degrees from good universities, followed by postgrad qualifications, and go on to edit national magazines. Nor do they have meaningful friendships and long marriages (my relationship may have ended but we gave it our best shot for 13 years).

The problem is that I am now looking back at my life to date and inventing deeply entrenched character flaws for myself. Yes, there were a couple of wobbles. When I was 18, I changed my undergraduate course from law to English, moving from Manchester to London, because I was unhappy. I missed my then-boyfriend, a photographer in the capital. But was this a sign of a fundamental defect in my sense of 'self'? I was a *baby*.

I was – I can't use the present tense any longer – an extrovert and could be impatient at times. But is this the definition of an Unstable Personality?

This diagnosis has me doubting myself and everything I have ever been. Perhaps my success was a fluke, my friendships an illusion. I am – and always have been – an imposter. It goes further: maybe I've never been a particularly nice person, deserving of love, or even capable of it.

If it was possible to feel worse than I did before, I now do. So, thanks, doctors and therapists.

When I question my diagnosis, I see looks being exchanged between professionals. The irony is that this makes me look even more Unstable. I feel like I am trapped in some Kafkaesque nightmare. But instead of waking up as a cockroach, I've been reincarnated as a long-stay psychiatric casualty.

NOTE: *Just writing this now from the future makes me feel angry on behalf of my younger, less resilient self. And a bit tearful, actually.*

I don't think either of these are unhealthy – or Emotionally Unstable – responses.

Personality disorders

A personality disorder is defined as 'a way of thinking, feeling and behaving that deviates from cultural expectations, causes distress or problems functioning, and lasts over time.'

'Everyone may feel emotional, get jealous, or want to be liked at times. But it is when these traits start to cause problems that you may be diagnosed as having a personality disorder,' says one mental health resource. 'You may find your emotions confusing, tiring, and hard to control. This can be distressing for you and others. Because it is distressing, you may find that you develop other mental health problems like depression or anxiety. You may also do other things such as drink heavily, use drugs, or self harm to cope.'

'All these symptoms can be linked to insomnia,' Dr Sophie Bostock tells me, today.

There are ten diagnosable personality disorders in the *DSM–V*, in three 'clusters':

Cluster A:

Paranoid Personality Disorder: You find yourself becoming suspicious of others without good reason.

Schizoid Personality Disorder: You are a loner with few social relationships and can appear cold.

Schizotypal Personality Disorder: You exhibit strange thoughts and behaviours and seem 'odd'.

Cluster B:

Antisocial Personality Disorder: You are impulsive, reckless, can be prone to violence and have little or no empathy.

Emotionally Unstable Personality Disorder (formerly known as Borderline Personality Disorder, BPD): Has a special entry of its own, see overleaf.

Histrionic Personality Disorder: You like being the centre of attention and are overly dramatic.

Narcissistic Personality Disorder: You feel entitled, self-important and do not acknowledge the feelings or needs of others.

Cluster C:

Dependent Personality Disorder: You allow others to take control of your life and have little self-confidence to act by yourself.

Avoidant Personality Disorder: You have a fear of being judged and feel uncomfortable in social situations.

Obsessive Personality Disorder: Characterized by a need for extreme perfection, order and neatness. Differs from obsessive compulsive disorder (OCD) because sufferers think their behaviour is reasonable and everyone else is 'wrong'.

In my personality disorder Google period, I became convinced I had every single one of these conditions, except possibly the last (which at least would have had the side effect of a tidy house).

For the purposes of this book, I am going to concentrate on **Emotionally Unstable Personality Disorder (EUPD)**, or BPD, because that, for a while, was my fate.

Personality disorder (PD) is a controversial diagnosis. In a 2013 blog for goodtherapy.org, psychotherapist Stacey Freedenthal wrote: 'The diagnosis of Borderline Personality Disorder carries profound stigma for many people. Even some mental health professionals use the term pejoratively – which is not difficult considering that the diagnosis itself implies that someone's personality is flawed. In reality, the flaw lies within the diagnosis.'

Dr Sami Timimi, our enlightened consultant NHS psychiatrist, says: 'When I was at medical school, we used to play a game. There were six people in our student house and we'd sit around, trying to work out which personality disorder category our housemates fell into.

'PD is an awful diagnosis. It's a bit like astrology: you pick the symptoms that suit your purposes.

'PD tends to be slapped on a patient if they a) don't get better and b) are seen as a pain in the neck by the team that is treating them. The mental health and psychiatry specialism has expanded since the closure of the asylums in the 1980s. Hence, with more long-term patients in community care, a PD diagnosis has become far more common.

'The patient is no longer seen as having an illness they can recover from. It's as though their whole being is discounted.

'A minority of patients welcome a PD diagnosis. They see it as an explanation for the difficulties they've been going through. But many of those then find it a dissatisfying pathway because having this label doesn't really solve anything.

'Other patients see it as a stigma; it makes them feel worse.

'It's also – as with much else in psychiatry – a subjective diagnosis. Who is the arbiter of what is "normal"? There is no discussion about parameters in this specialism. To illustrate: there is an anti-psychiatry movement but no anti-cardiology movement. Kidneys don't sit around and have dreams or anxiety about the future.

'Many mental health practitioners have an anxiety about dealing with distress and "otherness", so they dredge up this pseudo-diagnosis and hope the patient will go away. It deflects responsibility from the failure of treatment.

'There is also a gender divide in PD diagnoses: most with Antisocial Personality Disorder are men – which leads us into the whole "mad or bad?" debate. Seventy-five per cent of those diagnosed with EUPD are women. I see this as another way for the male-dominated adult world to pathologize the incredible demands made on women by society.

'Treatment for PD is limited on the NHS. The NICE guidelines tell doctors to avoid medication unless there is the coexistence of another condition. But given that nine out of ten people diagnosed are already on a cocktail of drugs, that's pretty difficult to follow.

'No one style of therapy is shown to be more effective than another, although dialectical behavioural therapy (DBT) is quite fashionable. DBT is based on cognitive behavioural therapy but it's specially adapted for people who feel emotions very intensely.

'DBT looks at ways of dealing with past trauma, among other things. But not everyone likes this approach: some patients would rather concentrate on their family relationships or not look back at all. There is no magic "cure".

'As a doctor, I am concerned about psychiatric labels. If an emotionally upset patient comes to see me, I view them as having a human experience first and foremost. Respecting the diversity of our reactions to life challenges means that the people I meet are nearly always reacting in ways that are "ordinary" and/or "understandable". A diagnosis can obscure this with potentially disastrous consequences.

'Every encounter has its unique aspects and each patient – or their family – develops a particular relationship with me. I want to know what they hope to achieve from the appointment and how things might look different if matters improved. Then I try to get my patients to visualize that.

'I want to get behind that initial "why?" question. If you understood why, what difference would that make in your real life? I usually do a genogram to see who is in the family, who lives with whom, etc., and what their broader social support network is. I want to understand their "resilience" towards other problems they've faced and how they dealt with them. I'm always on the lookout for these inner strengths that we regularly miss.

'Finally, I want to understand their "theory of change". How do they imagine change will happen? If they say it's medication I ask them to break this down into smaller steps of what they think they would first see and how that would affect others.

'If a patient disagrees with me I don't diagnose them with a PD. Rather, I welcome it as a quality of mental strength because most people find it hard to question their doctors.

'In practical terms, having a PD diagnosis on your medical records can hold you back in life: you may not be treated as seriously by your doctors as someone without this diagnosis.'

I think Dr Sami Timimi is a rather good psychiatrist. I wish I had visited his hospital.

NOTE: *I saw a number of consultant psychiatrists in subsequent years. Each told me that this diagnosis of EUPD was in error. But it was only after my interview with Dr Timimi that I thought to check whether the label had been removed from my current medical records. It hadn't.*

I'm happy to say that my GP listened to my concerns, read through the most recent correspondence on my mental health and struck the diagnosis off my medical history.

I am now – once again – officially the owner of a Stable Personality.

15th March

0 HOURS, 0 MINUTES

At some point, I am assigned a care coordinator, a kind of social worker who visits me at home from time to time, advising on benefits and overseeing the general welfare of the family. The personnel changes a couple of times. Every month or so, the current care coordinator and I sit in the living room – the conversation is the usual carousel of 'I can't sleep's and an exasperated/placatory response with vague promises to sort out 'a medication review' with my consultant.

(I remember one care coordinator getting a parking ticket. 'Crap!' she exclaimed. I filed this away for a time when such a thing might amuse me, which I think might be now.)

Otherwise, I don't recall much therapy beyond an assessment for something called a 'Welcome Group'. I assail the assessors with my insomniac desperation. The session ends in an immediate referral to an unfamiliar psychiatrist down the corridor and an emergency sleeping pill prescription on top of my benzos.

It doesn't work.

I do my own research. The neighbouring health authority has some sort of programme for those of disordered personality. But I live three streets in the wrong direction and can't access it.

On I plod with the clonazepam, the TV and twice-weekly visits to my private therapist who tries his very best to fix the damage done to my psyche by the NHS.

2nd April

0 HOURS, 0 MINUTES

Diagnoses fly around but still I can't sleep.

I have a new favourite thing on talkSPORT. 'Fisherman's Blues' is on weekend mornings at the crack of dawn. It's a show about catching trout and salmon but I have a strange attraction to it. The Waterboys' theme tune takes me back to student days.

13th May

MAYBE 20 MINUTES?

I'm in serious trouble with the clonazepam now. As my brain and body have become dependent, I need more pills to achieve that pleasant fuzziness. My doctor wisely only prescribes me a week at a time. Hence, I take extra, run out early and by the end of the weekend, I am desperate.

Surely it isn't normal to be jumping from foot to foot on a Monday morning, waiting for the chemist to open? I am terrified of the pharmacist turning up even ten minutes late. When she does unlock the shop door, she refuses to meet my eye (or maybe I'm just being paranoid). Either way, I feel ashamed of being a 'junkie'.

I revisit benzos on Google.

You are only supposed to be on them for a maximum of four weeks 'intermittently, if possible'. I have been on them for over 30 months. And constantly, not intermittently.

1st June

0 HOURS, 0 MINUTES

I ask my GP for help. She looks concerned but says she can only follow the directions of the consultant, who is, after all, a specialist. So, I start to research self-help websites.

In the forums and chat rooms are scary stories of people (mainly women) who have been on these drugs for years. Many are psychologically – some even physically – disabled as a result of taking benzos, which, I read to my additional joy, can raise the risk of cancer or nerve damage. There are a number of helplines on the net but every time I call, I get an answerphone message.

Eventually, someone calls me back. I am directed to an online resource called *The Ashton Manual*. This is a programme written in 1999 by pharmacologist Professor Heather Ashton which details a routine by which you gradually cut down your benzo use over a long period of time until you eventually 'jump off'.

This certainly makes sense in theory. But do I have the mental strength/desire to do it right now?

On Heather Ashton and *The Ashton Manual*

Heather Ashton was a physician and a British emeritus professor of clinical psychopharmacology at Newcastle University. In the mid-1980s, she started to publish papers on the adverse effects of long-term use of benzodiazepines and the problems of withdrawal. Ashton wrote 50 such studies in all.

She developed an approach to withdrawal that supported the patient to take over their own treatment and control the rate at which their medication was lowered, in small but carefully controlled doses. Ashton recommended that patients switch from stronger benzos such as lorazepam or temazepam to a 'weaker' benzo with a longer half life, usually diazepam (Valium).

On Professor Ashton's clock, complete withdrawal would take months – even years. In 1999, she distilled her experience into a manual, *Benzodiazepines: How They Work and How to Withdraw*. Such was the demand for *The Ashton Manual* – as it came to be known – that it has since appeared in 11 languages and several updated editions, all available to download for free.

Professor Ashton's views were initially challenged by some psychiatrists. However, by the late 1990s, most accepted that long-term use of benzodiazepines was not safe.

Because of widespread prescribing and easy availability, Professor Ashton was one of the first people to comment when benzodiazepines entered the 'street' drug scene. In the 2001 foreword to *The Ashton Manual*, she stated:

'They are taken illicitly in high doses by 90 per cent of polydrug abusers world-wide, unleashing new and dangerous effects (AIDS, hepatitis, and risks to the next generation) which were undreamt of when benzos were introduced into medicine as a harmless panacea nearly 50 years ago.'

Following an appeal from the British Medical Association, in 2013 the British National Formulary revised its guide-lines on withdrawal to align with the latest edition of *The Ashton Manual*.

Millions of patients worldwide since benefited from these changes in practice.

When Professor Ashton died in September 2019, she was mourned far and wide.

But, life gets worse when you try to come off the bloody benzos . . .

In her book, *A Straight Talking Introduction to Psychiatric Drugs: The Truth About How They Work and How to Come Off Them*, Professor Joanna Moncrieff states:

'Benzodiazepine withdrawal reactions are well recognized and include a huge variety of symptoms. Since they are nervous system depressants, stopping them increases the sensitivity of the nervous system. Therefore withdrawal symptoms commonly include anxiety, agitation, insomnia and mood swings. Unpleasant sensory experiences such as tingling and numbness, pain and electric-shock-like feelings in the head can occur.'

Professor Moncrieff goes on to list these further symptoms:

- tinnitus (ringing sounds in the ear)
- depersonalization (feeling 'unreal')
- heightened sensitivity to light, noise or touch
- muscle spasms, stiffness and tics
- flu-like symptoms: sweating and shivering
- loss of appetite
- depression
- increased heart rate and blood pressure

Need I go on?

Yes! 'Since benzodiazepines have anti-epileptic properties, rapid withdrawal can cause dangerous epileptic fits.'

8th June

0 HOURS, 0 MINUTES

Enough, I tell myself. You made a mistake by going on these pills, you can damn well come off them. But I do need some help. I take myself to the local drug and alcohol service, a walk-in clinic based at the nearby hospital. I don't care that I am in a waiting room with people who clearly have serious substance abuse issues.

That very afternoon, I see a counsellor and am referred to see a consultant who specializes in treating addicts. Addict. Yep, it's a loaded word but that's what I am now. I need to get used to it.

Addicted or dependent? The politics

So, this is a tricky area. When I started writing newspaper articles about my problems with prescription drugs, I talked about my 'addiction'. Certain online patients' groups jumped on me for using this word.

They drew a difference between iatrogenic dependence – 'relating to illness caused by medical examination or treatment' – and 'street' addiction.

'We are not addicts,' they said. 'Addicts are people who choose to take drugs recreationally, for their own pleasure. We were given these medications by our doctors. We didn't abuse them. Please can you use the word "dependent" in future?'

So, which is correct? And does it matter?

Dr Mark Horowitz is a training psychiatrist/research fellow at University College London and doughty campaigner against the overprescription of harmful psychiatric medications. He says:

'Dependence and addiction are often confused – but the distinction between the two is important because they are treated differently medically.

'Dependence is a physical process, which is why it is often called physical dependence or physiological dependence. It happens whenever anyone uses a dependence-inducing substance. The body becomes used to the substance through a physical process (for example, reduced number of receptors). If someone is dependent on a substance, then they will get withdrawal symptoms if they reduce or stop that substance.

'Addiction is a condition where the reward system in the brain is hijacked by a substance and involves: impaired control over drug use, compulsive use (using whenever there is access to the drug), continued use despite harm (job loss, relationship breakdown) and craving (wanting the drug when they cannot have it).

'You can see that this is different from someone who is prescribed a drug like a benzodiazepine by their doctor. They take the drug because they have been told it is a useful treatment to take – and they follow their doctor's orders. Anyone who takes a dependence-forming drug for long enough (often a few weeks) will become dependent on it to some degree and many will have a hard time stopping because of withdrawal symptoms.

'Many will also experience "tolerance": the need for a higher dose to get the same effect. This happens commonly with benzodiazepines. They may also get "inter-dose withdrawal" where they start to get withdrawal symptoms in the time in between doses as the effect on the body has started to wear off more quickly.

'Of course, all people with any sort of drug-related issue deserve help. However, there are many drug and alcohol services in England for people who are addicted to substances. But there are currently no specialized services for people who have become involuntarily dependent on a prescribed drug. Most of these people were not told that these drugs – benzodiazepines, 'Z-drugs', gabapentinoids (see page 209) and, it's now becoming clear, antidepressants – are dependence-forming. Many do not think it is appropriate to be sent to addiction services for medications that they took as prescribed by their doctors.

'Because of a stigma attached to addiction, sometimes when people who are dependent on a medication tell their doctor that they cannot stop because of withdrawal symptoms, they are told that they must have become addicted (i.e. are misusing the drug in some way) and that doctors shouldn't prescribe to addicts. Some people then find that the doctor refuses to prescribe for an 'addict' and find themselves in the dire position of being unable to get a prescription for the drug they are now involuntarily dependent on. They must then find another doctor, who might look at them suspiciously: "why are you seeing a new doctor to get a script for Valium?".

'If this is seen as "weakness of character" then these people are not given the help they need but sometimes treated punitively, or offered addiction classes so they can try to overcome their "addiction".

'Benzodiazepines can cause dependence (in all people who take them for a significant period of time) and addiction (in a small minority). Most people understand that it would be inappropriate to send granny to the local addiction service if she can't sleep when she stops her sleeping pills, or give her a stern talking to about her problem being addicted to sleeping pills.'

This is powerful stuff, which I only discovered as I was coming to the close of writing this book. I have an awful lot of sympathy for the correct use of terminology here, especially if it could change the treatment pathway of a person with a prescription drug dependency.

But I also feel strongly that people who have problems with alcohol or street drugs are no 'worse' than those who got their pills from doctors, though our treatment should be different (see page 130). For sure, 'dependent' sounds like the better way to describe my state at this time, but I was soon to be in Rehab Land, where the lingo is soundly that of 'addiction'.

So, with heartfelt apologies to those who strongly advocate the use of 'dependence' – and I totally get where you are coming from – for the following pages, I will continue to talk about my 'addiction' to benzodiazepines.

14th June

O HOURS, O MINUTES

I meet the addictions consultant. We agree I will taper the clonazepam à la *Ashton Manual* and switch to diazepam, which is a milder, longer-acting benzo.

Hence, the plan is that I will cut it down to smaller and smaller doses over a matter of months until the drug is safely out of my system.

It is dangerous to go 'cold turkey' because it can lead to seizures, which could potentially be fatal. This cannot be repeated enough, people.

The large amounts of clonazepam I'm taking translate to 50mg of Valium. That is a *lot*.

But the plan could work and, with some professional support, I feel emboldened to try.

What an odd situation this is. I am seeing a doctor to discuss ways to come off a drug while, two floors up, in the same building, lurks the doctor who put me on it in the first place.

30th June

O HOURS, O MINUTES

I return to the unit for a follow-up. As I'm leaving, a friendly psych patient calls out: 'Hello, Amy Winehouse!' All I have in common with sadly departed Amy are Jewish-ish looks, my stress-and-sleeplessness-related weight loss and the little dress and skinny jeans I am wearing.

But there are the pills, of course. The irony does not escape me.

1st July

O HOURS, O MINUTES

The addictions consultant is sympathetic but I feel I need extra support coming off such a large whack of diazepam.

And Internet advice is all very well but what I really need is an actual person to speak to, a dedicated counsellor, maybe. The problem is, expert help seems almost non-existent. I discover charities in random places like Bristol and Oldham. Then – hurrah! – I find there is another, just down the road from me. I call the number and amazingly get through to someone straight away. The woman is kind, but regretful. If you live outside this particular borough then they can't help. You are not eligible.

I am surprised, annoyed and frustrated. I can't be the only person with this problem. Why is there not more provision out there to help me? What do others in my situation do?

15th July

O HOURS, O MINUTES

In the end, Anthony, my therapist, throws up his hands, says he has done everything he can but is powerless to help me. Not only is he failing to make a difference but his impotence is starting to affect his own sense of wellbeing.

With heavy hearts on both sides, we agree to stop the sessions.

I will never forget Anthony's kindnesses. In the future, we will become friends who have lunch from time to time and set the world to rights.

26th September

O HOURS, O MINUTES

In a follow-up appointment, I tell my original psychiatrist that I'm worried about the amount of benzos I'm taking, and that I'm trying to cut down.

'OK,' he says, 'but let's also try something else.' He takes out his British National Formulary and puts me on a small dose of a newish drug called pregabalin, which he says could be phased in as a replacement and isn't addictive. *The Ashton Manual* doesn't come up.

Oh well, more to the party.

5th October

O HOURS, O MINUTES

Back on Google, I am rereading – with my customary obsession – the websites about long-term benzo use and the problems this can cause. I decide that all my problems are down to my dependence on these drugs. Twisted logic in my brain tells me that if I 'normalize' my brain chemistry, I might 'reset' and start to sleep again.

I'm just too weak to keep going by myself. So, maybe I'll pay some professionals to do it for me.

I start to look for rehab units that offer help for prescription drug addicts. (NHS in-patient help seems practically non-existent. Units seem to be mainly for alcoholics and heroin addicts, and look – quite frankly – scary.)

There is a dizzying array of private clinics and I really have no idea how to choose. I discount the silly-money ones in Arizona and those famously frequented by celebrities. One or two insist that 'clients' share rooms; I cross those off the list.

I make some calls. Some clinics admit they don't have the medical staff required to oversee my withdrawal safely but others enthusiastically report success in bringing people off benzos. One of these is not too expensive, is within striking distance of London and the staff sound friendly and experienced.

I (don't) sleep on it.

10th October

0 HOURS, 0 MINUTES

I call my chosen clinic and things happen very quickly. They send a car for me within two hours.

My driver is Z, a cheerful 20-something who tells me the clinic helped her recover from years of cocaine addiction. 'It's brilliant,' she says. 'We will get you well.'

It's exactly what I want to hear. 'We'. A team is going to swoop in and take over! They are going to sort me out!

We arrive at the suburb where the clinic is set. Clients are housed in blocks with a sort of 'house manager'. I'm shown to my 'house' and it's empty. 'They're all at a meeting,' says Z. I ask what kind of a meeting. 'Alcoholics Anonymous,' she says. 'You'll be joining them tomorrow.'

Really? But I'm not an alcoholic.

Z explains that all the meetings are compulsory and gives me some reading material. She takes my pills away and says the clinic GP is on her way. I also have to hand in my mobile phone – clients apparently get their phones back after the first week (and are then only allowed them in the evenings). This doesn't bother me in the least. Who am I going to call, anyway?

The doctor is young and understanding. She listens to my tale of woe. Together we draw up what sounds like a reasonable benzo reduction programme. Because I am in a supervised environment, she says we can go more quickly than if I was at home. We aim for three weeks, with one drug-free week at the end, so I'll make the most of the therapies on offer.

A standard rehab stay is 28 days and it all sounds pretty good to me.

Best of all, the GP gives me two zopiclones to take that night, so I get a good night in order to make the most of my introduction the next day.

Extra drugs at rehab? Bonus.

11th October

0 HOURS, 0 MINUTES

Early hours: But, of course, I don't sleep.

I read the literature that Z has given me. The clinic is set up around the '12-Step' programme. It's in the 'rules' that there are five meetings a week: a mix of AA and NA (Narcotics Anonymous). I ask myself how much any of this applies to me, then decide that I probably should have read the clinic's website properly before choosing it.

Caveat emptor.

I don't know much about the 12-Step programme, except that Robbie Williams praised it in some documentary for helping him to get sober. But I do recall that the 12 Steps are famous for helping millions of people across the world. So I decide to go with it and immerse myself in what the clinic has to offer. If nothing else, the meetings will be interesting.

Morning: Dazed with tiredness and a bit disorientated, I come downstairs to meet my housemates. I make an effort.

People are friendly. There is one other pale-faced new arrival who is coming off an alcohol binge and keeps rushing to the loo and a healthy-looking lady who tells me she has kicked her drink habit and is leaving that Friday.

Over breakfast, I'm encouraged to talk about why I am there. A chap in his late twenties tells me of his terrific experiences of taking handfuls of zopiclone (or zopis, as he calls them) during the day. I listen politely and offer my own tame story, which doesn't have quite the same bravado.

We then all head off to the 'clinic' some distance away.

Afternoon: I don't remember much. There is an awful lot to take in – hours of sitting on chairs in circles and hearing people read out their 'step work' from paper printouts they have filled in by hand. I am given 'Step One, Part One' as my first homework, in which I must acknowledge that my life has 'become unmanageable' and I am 'powerless over my poison' (benzos).

Easy! I admit it!

There are also therapy groups with different focuses – we watch a video on the origins of addiction as a disease, narrated for some reason by a man hiking through the Colorado desert.

It's all a bit discombobulating.

Evening: The housemates take turns to cook. (If this sounds like *Big Brother*, well, you wouldn't be a million miles off.) An Indian woman makes an amazing curry.

Over dinner, I ask whether anyone has experience with benzos. Blank faces: most people have never heard of them. A couple of my fellow diners with alcohol problems have actually been *put on* weak doses of a benzo called Librium to help with their detoxes. But no one has these drugs as a primary problem. Nor have they come across anyone else – either currently in treatment or a recent leaver – who has.

The house manager says she recalls 'one person, earlier this year' who has and will investigate further for me.

I am not encouraged.

Then everyone has 20 minutes to get ready for an NA meeting. I am so exhausted and overwhelmed, I beg the house manager to *please* let me off going. I sense a hint of disapproval but she makes a call and I am 'allowed' to stay home because I am new. From tomorrow, I have to attend.

12th October

0 HOURS, 0 MINUTES

There is an interesting mix of people in rehab.

There is no 'type'. I meet: an older woman from Scotland who drinks a bottle of vodka a day; a PR with tattoos and a ruby-pierced nipple (she shows me), also an alcoholic; a fireman who is an alcoholic; a young, trust-fundy guy who has problems with ketamine; an executive coke-head; a heroin addict who has been back many times and looks like he'll probably be back again.

Almost all of them are very nice. The tattooed PR lends me her beauty products and tries to tame my wild, wiry curls with olive oil spray.

But try as I might, I just don't 'get' discussions around drug and alcohol use, nor do I identify with their 'journeys'.

Rehab – or this particular rehab – is quite 'hard knocks', from the counsellors down to the residents and the former clients who help out with driving, etc.

I, on the other hand, am a wuss.

The 12-Step programme

Originally part of the Alcoholics Anonymous movement, the 12 Steps are a programme charting a course of action for 'recovery' with the goal of becoming 'clean' or 'sober'.

The 12 Steps were first published in the 1939 book *Alcoholics Anonymous: The Story of How More Than One Hundred Men Have Recovered from Alcoholism* by William G Wilson. He is usually referred to as 'Bill W', and the book is nicknamed 'the Big Book'.

The AA method was adapted and became the foundation of other 12-step programmes for other substances including drugs and later for behavioural problems such as sex or even shopping.

Some people start their 12-Step experience in rehab. Many others go straight to 'meetings', such as AA and NA. These are often held in church halls and community centres, or, these days, on Zoom. There is tea, coffee and biscuits.

The 12 Steps is the inspiration behind and the backbone of these gatherings, where fellow addicts share their experiences, celebrate each other's sobriety and support those who have 'relapsed'. There is usually an inspirational speaker, who is 'in recovery'. The aim is 'spiritual awakening' and to learn from the struggles and triumphs of others.

People get coloured 'sobriety chips': round bits of plastic with numbers on to celebrate a period of abstinence.

The 12 Steps can be found on the Alcoholics Anonymous website (see Resources on page 283). They are a kind of 'ladder' of 'recovery' that begins with admitting one has a problem, all the way up to having a 'spiritual awakening' and helping other people overcome their own issues with addiction. On this journey, addicts are encouraged to do certain things, such as making 'a fearless moral inventory of ourselves', and to promise to make amends to those they've hurt. The words 'God', 'Higher Power' and 'prayer' feature prominently.

Nicky Walton-Flynn is an addictions therapist who advocates the 12 Steps.

She says: 'The 12-Step programme is a spiritual philosophy and a way of living a kind life. Its aim is to offer clients empowerment, love, the capacity for behavioural change and, most importantly, hope. Without hope, you don't get up.

'I see it as a similar model to CBT.

'Those who endorse the Steps feel that addiction is not just a physical dependency (though it can be that, too) but a way of thinking. My favourite definition is that it's "a pathological relationship with a substance or a behaviour" which achieves the buzz of feel-good brain chemicals such as dopamine or endorphins. An addict keeps repeating this behaviour, even though the "intelligent" side knows it's bad for them.

'I know that people struggle with the religious implications of "Higher Power". I tell them to imagine a person or a place where they feel a sense of peace. It could be God in the traditional sense but also a wise grandmother, a quiet woodland, even astrophysics.

'Some people work on the 12 Steps alone or with a therapist such as myself. But there is also the Fellowship – groups such as AA or CA (Cocaine Anonymous) where people can be around others they identify with. These groups transcend class and intellect and offer great support.

'Rehab becomes necessary when the person needs a medical withdrawal or has to be taken out of their environment because the stimuli and triggers that keep them addicted are too acute.'

NOTE: *There is no Benzos Anonymous.*

13th October

0 HOURS, 0 MINUTES

I'm staring at my Step One form. Yes, I'm powerless over benzos. My life is unmanageable, for sure. But why do I have to read from, and précis bits from, the Big Book?

It feels a bit like being back at school.

14th October

0 HOURS, 0 MINUTES

A day in rehab

9am: Off we head to the clinic, to the accompaniment of uplifting music. 'Feelin' Good' is a favourite. I am not feeling good because I have not slept a wink, and actually wish people would keep their optimism to themselves, thanks.

9.30am: On arrival at the clinic, we scramble to pick up pieces of paper left on the floor in the middle of the room. We are supposed to record our thoughts and feelings. I can't get beyond: 'I didn't sleep again.' Then there is a 'gratitude' list – we have to write five things we are grateful for. I can't think of one.

10am: *Just for Today* is the addicts' bible: a book of spiritual, uplifting homilies. We are each supposed to read one out and are encouraged to find meaning in our portions. People recite, impressively reflect and talk about their personal progress. I struggle to even do the first part of this. The blurry words dance in front of my eyes. I read on a blank autopilot, without any attempt at insight beyond pale platitudes.

The truth is that, unlike everyone else in the room, I am not progressing. In fact, as the withdrawal symptoms of my detox start to kick in, I feel steadily worse.

In the end, I feel so self-conscious about not recovering, I start making up positive comments.

This session always ends with the Serenity Prayer:

'God grant me the serenity
to accept the things I cannot change;
courage to change the things I can;
and wisdom to know the difference.'

I happen to think the Serenity Prayer is beautiful and wise. But I'm not really a fan of standing in a circle holding hands, nor the sort of 'group hug' element to the whole thing.

There is a lot of 'group hugginess' in rehab.

11am: Meditation. A skilled therapist takes the 30-minute meditation session. We are encouraged to close our eyes, follow her creative visualizations and chill. It's similar to the progressive relaxations I tried right back at the start of my Insomnia Crash.

The grave silence of meditation is not helped by the sound of a delivery lorry, which arrives at exactly the same time every morning, playing loud music like an ice-cream van. It rather jars with the babbling brooks and deserted beaches.

Despite my ongoing distress, I always want to snigger at this point. I squint my eyes open to see if anyone else feels the same, but everyone is earnestly drifting away down a flowing river.

At the end, the therapist 'brings us back'. Everyone stretches, grins and says how amazing that was, how relaxed they feel.

I am so tense, I can feel my teeth grinding together. My muscles are locked and achy. It doesn't occur to me that this might be down to the benzo withdrawals.

Step meetings: Every three days or so, each person takes a turn to present their paperwork. The assembled company listens respectfully. The group leader makes some initial comments, then others are encouraged to pitch in.

You get a 'pass' or a 'fail'. I fly through the easy Step One, Part One, but I fail Part Two.

'What does being an addict mean to you?' reads the question. I write – and read out to the assembled company – a carefully written statement that I am ashamed, that this wasn't what I set out to become, that I had always worked hard and done my best. I am humbled and now realize that I am no 'better' than someone who has drunk to excess or chosen the path of street drugs.

WRONG ANSWER! I am told that I need to have quoted something from Bill's Big Book rather than given my visceral answer to this question.

I am put on the rehab naughty step and told to go away and do my 'step work' again.

Lunch: I am invariably relieved when we break for a sandwich lunch, prepared that morning by the inmates. But, uncertain of my place in this company, and not fitting into any of the cliques, I sit on my own and overeat.

The best part of lunch break is a walk through the nearby forest. One of the more seasoned peers is instructed to 'take care' of me and shepherd me safely through the woods.

We don't say much to one another but I am grateful for this gesture.

Afternoon session: This is similar to the morning. When business is concluded, we have timetabled chores which include hoovering the meeting room and cleaning up the small kitchen.

Then, back home for dinner and an hour or so's R and R.

Evening meetings: We pile into a minibus we call the 'Druggy Buggy' (ha!) and off to NA or AA meetings in the local area. I always do my best to get out of these. No dice. My presence is required.

The evening journeys to and from the meetings are a chance for hearty hilarity among my peers. One guy talks about drinking hand sanitizer in A&E and everyone commiserates.

I learn that there is a thing called 'euphoric recall', when addicts remember the great times they had on their substances of choice before it all went to shit. Euphoric recall is not encouraged but there is a lot of it on these minibus journeys.

I can't join in. As we top a hill on 5th November and see fireworks exploding everywhere, I have never felt more alone in my life.

5th November

O HOURS, O MINUTES

I am not making the expected progress, and so it is agreed my stay in rehab should be extended beyond the standard 28 days.

6th November

O HOURS, O MINUTES

Some of the 12 Steps make an awful lot of common sense. There is a saying that particularly stays with me: 'Keep your side of the street clean'. In other words, be responsible for your own good behaviour. It's a good rule for life. I like the notion that resentment is unhelpful and that you should make amends (where possible) to people you have hurt through your addiction.

But there is quite a lot of new age-y wafflespeak in AA. People swear by the Affirmations, which are things like: 'I am the boss of me.'

I am not a fan of this sort of stuff. These phrases are – to me – meaningless platitudes.

Most of all, I have problems with the 'Higher Power', in whom one's salvation is invested. I just don't buy it. Try as the counsellors might to insist that it's not religious – that your Higher Power can be your late grandpa or a child-hood pet – I just don't like the God-squad connotations that still linger from AA's 1930s Christian origins.

It all feels very conservative America and a bit 'culty'.

Year Ten: A note from the future

Reading back, I realize that I sound like a snob.

I do apologize if I offend any readers who have or have had problems with alcohol or recreational drugs and have been helped by 12-step programmes. I am learning that these problems are, of course, to be taken seriously and can result from a lifetime's trauma and unhappiness.

But the point is that – rather than feeling superior to the rest of the gang at the time – I felt quite the opposite.

I was such a loser, I even failed at rehab.

8th November

O HOURS, O MINUTES

As the weeks go by, my medication dose is lowered.

And every day, I feel worse and worse.

I feel antsy, deranged. I can't sit still, moving from place to place, room to room, running up and down the stairs. I can't concentrate on my chores.

I just can't 'be' with myself. I believe the word for this state is 'agitation' but that doesn't do it credit. It's like an unbearable psychic itchiness.

But I do have the self-awareness to see I am starting to be seen as a 'difficult' client: failing my step work, doing my cleaning jobs really badly, trying to get out of AA meetings.

I talk to R, one of the counsellors, a leopard print-clad former Rock chick and a woman I really like. I tell her that I'm not trying to be awkward but I feel physically terrible. I am really struggling, here.

R listens with some sympathy but says my addiction is the same as everyone else's, just a 'different poison'. She tells me an awful story about coming off heroin and speedballs cold turkey (for the uninitiated: speedballs are a mixture of cocaine and heroin. I am learning things).

When I talk about my kids and how guilty I feel, R commiserates, shares her experience and does make me feel better (briefly, temporarily).

But in the other daily groups, I can feel others' patience wearing thin. One group leader says that I am still in 'active addiction' and I should suspend my step work.

I know I am boring. I am reprimanded for being quiet. This therapist uses one 'circle time' to ask others what they think of me. The silence is deafening, despite the kind cocaine addict who ventures hesitantly: 'She's lovely.' (We have barely spoken, but I am grateful for his generosity.)

At the end of this session, the group leader makes me stand on a chair and sing 'God Save the Queen'. I think he's trying to use 'tough love' on me to bring me out of myself.

But I am mortified and tearful.

And I am *paying* for this.

That night: I study myself in the mirror.

I am thin and scraggy with terrible flaky skin. I don't bother with cosmetics – even moisturizer – and can't remember the last time I went out in the sun. My hair is dry. I've been using my husband's supermarket anti-dandruff shampoo and not bothering with conditioner.

If I put on lipstick, I look worse, like a benzo-addicted Joker.

I haven't bought any clothes for four years. Instead, I hang around in old leggings, a scruffy hoodie and some ancient down-at-heel Ugg boots. My next-door neighbour feels sorry for me and lends me some clothes. I pick up a few things at Primark on one of the Saturday outings to the local unprepossessing town.

What would Magazine Editor Miranda have thought of *that*?

But it's not just the physical, of course. I have gone from a successful, creative wife, mother and friend, to a lonely drug-addled spectre.

Yet I am being made to feel guilty and ashamed.

I don't morally judge the alcoholics and recreational drug users. In fact, since arriving at rehab, my eyes have been opened to some terrible life stories that I would never have otherwise encountered in my privileged middle-class bubble. I see that most people are generally decent and coping the best way they can, even if they sometimes make some bad choices.

But despite all of this: IT'S NOT *FAIR*.

10th November

O HOURS, O MINUTES

Morning: I tell the assembled addicts that I'm going to try coming off the pregabalin as well.

'Gabba gabba,' echoes the group leader, taking the piss.

Everyone falls about laughing. Again, I am humiliated.

Evening: A concerned alcoholic sees me pacing aimlessly outside a meeting and offers me a cigarette. I light it. Perhaps I should just try to fit in a bit more. (I am not very good at smoking either and cough a bit.)

At AA, I say, 'My name's Miranda and I'm an alcoholic.' It's a mix of resigned and passive-aggressive behaviour but I just don't give a shit any more.

My thoughts turn again to suicide and I share my anguish on my daily update form. Before I know it, I am hauled upstairs to the staff room. It feels like I'm being summoned to the headmaster's office.

A committee of three interrogates me. They are not able to cope with suicidal people, they say, they may have to discharge me.

But I don't want to leave. I don't want to go 'home' – in fact, I'm not even sure I have a home any longer. I tell the counsellors that I'm really sorry, I didn't mean it and I won't do it again.

I am sent downstairs and do the walk of shame, interrupting a Step Group to take my place.

Patience is wearing thin, all around.

11th November

O HOURS, O MINUTES

The clinic and I sign an armistice and decide that it would be better if I leave the next day.

I think I am down to 15mg of Valium. The GP 'ups' me to 20mg, to be safe. Nothing is said about the pregabalin; it's just stopped.

I give up on the benzo withdrawal for now.

NOTE: *It's also dangerous to stop taking pregabalin suddenly. I was only on a small dose at this point, so somehow escaped the seizures and suicidal thoughts that can happen when you stop suddenly. See page 209 for more on pregabalin.*

Rehab – where did it all go wrong?

I go back to Nicky Walton-Flynn, the addictions therapist. Nicky says: 'It seems to me that this particular clinic was not equipped to take you on. You say you called other treatment centres who turned you down for this reason. They were the honest ones.

'"Tough love" was completely the wrong approach for you. It needed to be gentle. I don't think you were in any place to consider a Higher Power. If I were your therapist, I would ask you to conjure up one moment in your day where you might not have felt as bad: brushing your teeth, say, or waiting for the kettle to boil.

'Many addiction therapists promote the 12-Step model to the letter; often through their own personal experiences. I am an advocate of the programme, however, I strongly believe that it needs to be worked into a more integrative therapeutic approach, whereby the 12-Step/Big Book model is seen as a scaffolding upon which to build.

'It may not have been the right time for you to attempt the 12 Steps. This is a shame because it should be a programme built on kindness. So, what would I have advised if you had come to me? You clearly needed a longer physical detox than you had. If money were no object, I would have sent you off to a specialist clinic in the United States where stays are for several months.

'It makes me sad to see how little affordable provision there is for people coming off prescription drugs. The government is just not willing to put money behind this.'

Coming off benzos: what *should* happen?

The problem is that there are very few UK experts in this field. As I write, I am advised of one specialist centre in London, two in Bristol and one in Oldham. I find Melanie Davis, manager of the oldest specialist benzodiazepine service in London.

Melanie has worked with benzo-dependent individuals for more than 25 years. As well as helping clients in an organization called Change Grow Live REST Service (the REST stands for Recovery, Experience, Sleeping Pills and Tranquilisers), she sits on various parliamentary committees and the Council for Evidence-Based Psychiatry and has given advice to NICE and the British Medical Association.

What Melanie doesn't know about benzos could be balanced on the top of a lorazepam. She even sets benzo quizzes for GPs. Benzo quizzes!

I wish I had known Melanie during my Insomnia Crash.

Melanie says: 'Benzodiazepines are distinct compounds and cannot be treated in the same way as other addictive substances. They need separate attention.

'"Regular" rehab is often not appropriate and most rehab workers do not have specialist training in this area.

'Benzo addiction is not "sexy". One of the first problems is that people tend to think they are benign, little-old-lady drugs from the sixties. The tag: "Mother's Little Helper" – as in the Rolling Stones' song – really doesn't help. I sometimes used to see a particular client in the supermarket. You wouldn't imagine there was anything wrong with her, but she was on 300mg of Valium a day. That is an enormous amount and the highest quantity I have come across anyone taking. She got them from a private prescription.

'Some of our clients are illicit drug users – the American drug Xanax is a modern problem. Then there are those who initially came to the services with an alcohol addiction, were put on benzos to help them come off and, 30 years on, are still on the benzos. Regardless of someone's pathway into dependency, we offer support.

'The majority of our clients are long-term prescription users who went to their GPs in good faith. Clients range from 18 to 87, with an average age of 55. Forty per cent are male and sixty per cent are female.

'Doctors vastly underestimate the problems caused by these drugs.

'"Addicted or dependent"? I prefer "involuntarily dependent".

'The problems of being on benzos long-term include: emotional blunting (the inability to "feel"), feelings of panic, agoraphobia, blurry vision and brain fog. Interactions with alcohol make all of this worse. Dependency is a huge issue. Go on holiday without your benzos and you will probably have to fly home again.

'When perfectly respectable people are cut off from their script, they will go "doctor shopping" to find a GP who will prescribe them, or turn to the Internet, or even street dealers.

'You can't come off benzos suddenly. If you do, you could have a fatal seizure.

'This is one of the reasons why the 12-Step programme – which can be life-saving for other addictions – is not appropriate. It is based on abstinence: you have to stop and stay stopped, which you can't do suddenly with a benzo.

'There is no Benzos Anonymous for precisely this reason. Some sufferers find the religious overtones of the Fellowship a bit inflexible. REST offers a user-centred, "mutual aid" approach.

'Even if you don't go cold turkey (and this really is dangerous), you need to avoid a too-rapid withdrawal. Without a medically supervised taper, people coming off could suffer with something called protracted withdrawal syndrome (see page 143).

'Problems could last for years. They include terrible sleep difficulties, anxiety, depression and flu-like symptoms.'

How Melanie treats someone with a benzo problem:

- 'Two things need to be addressed: the pharmacological dependency and the psychological one. A skilled thera-pist knows that the two are linked.
- With the help of the client's GP, I will work out a daily prescription. Say you are taking 30mg of Valium a day and occasionally dabble with 50mg – we will try to stick at 30mg. Then we aim for a slow taper along with therapy and support.

- The more gradual the reduction, the better. How much we "jump down" depends very much on the client's age, circumstances, how long they have taken benzodiazepines for and what they feel is achievable.

'We offer groups for people to support each other and share their experiences, moderated by experienced volunteers and formal counselling.'

What to do if you are dependent on benzodiazepines and want to stop:

- 'DO NOT STOP SUDDENLY.
- If you feel your use/withdrawal has become a medical emergency, call the emergency services.
- Benzo dependency can be a very lonely place. Enlist the support of friends and family if you can.
- If you are lucky enough to be in an area that offers specialist benzo support, make an appointment to see an adviser.
- Try one of the few existing helplines, to be found on the Internet, or see Resources on page 283.
- I would highly advise looking up *The Ashton Manual* (see page 103). Stabilize your dose; do not go any days without your tablets.
- Educate yourself on your condition. Specialist web-sites and their forums can be helpful. Don't take too much notice of the horror stories, however. Every person is different and if you handle your withdrawal responsibly, you may not need to suffer unnecessarily.
- Local NHS drug and alcohol services can be useful, especially if you need help with housing, finances, child custody, etc.

- Hold on to your own identity. Remember who you were before your current problems and aim to be that person again.
- Eat well and exercise if you can. But it can be really difficult to motivate yourself physically, both when on benzos and coming off them. Be realistic: some people can head off on ten-kilometre cycle rides but most cannot.
- Do try to get out of the house every day. This can be easier said than done: agoraphobia is a common side effect of benzo use and withdrawal.
- Go easy on yourself: it's a tough old job coming off these drugs. Some clients who have also used other substances report that they are the hardest drugs to withdraw from.
- Remember, there is hope! In the vast majority of cases, the damage is not permanent – new neural pathways are being created all the time. I have not worked with one client who didn't improve, to some degree.'

What needs to happen, according to Melanie:

'The government should provide services for iatrogenic addiction. GPs and psychiatrists need to receive up-to-date education in the dangers of these drugs and specialist training in how to take people off them.'

Melanie knows it all! She gets it!

12th November

0 HOURS, 0 MINUTES

Two counsellors from the clinic drive me back to London. I ask them to drop me at A&E. Maybe a 'normal' NHS psychiatric admission is what I need. Perhaps there is a miracle drug for sleep that people have been keeping from me. Or some understanding of the whole benzo withdrawal mess.

The counsellors take me to the emergency department at my local hospital and run.

I spend another day in one of those rooms with the blue plastic chairs. Next to me is a large bag containing everything I took with me to rehab. It's pretty much all the clothing I have these days. I feel like a homeless person.

Eventually, one of the A&E psychiatric team arrives. She doesn't know what to do with me, either.

It's very hard to land a place at a psychiatric unit – and even rarer that people turn up and ask to be admitted. But someone, somewhere, senses my desperation and a bed is found. I imagine I'll be carted off to the local unit I visited as an outpatient but there is no room at the inn.

Hence, I am destined for somewhere else, in an unfamiliar part of the city. NHS mental patients don't get to pick and choose. En route, the ambulance swoops past the end of my road.

I panic. I want to get off!

Even though I now believe I am making a terrible mistake, I am so paralysed, I don't say anything to the paramedics. (Though I hardly think they would say 'OK, then', and drop me at my front door.) Instead, we arrive in the dead of night at a gloomy, long, low building.

Sticky double doors lock behind me as I enter the ward and am shown to my 'room', which is a curtained-off part of a ward of six, barely two metres wide.

What am I *doing*?

13th November

MINUS 2 HOURS. IS THAT POSSIBLE?

At 2am, someone in the curtained-off cubicle opposite me starts singing in an unfamiliar language. I ask them to please keep it down but they pretend not to hear me. Before I have time to complain to the manager the next day, I am transferred to my local hospital.

Now, I am a big fan of the NHS. And I wish I didn't have to trot out the same tired clichés about the appalling state of mental health provision in this country. But, sadly, I have no choice. I was not a big fan of being an NHS psychiatric in-patient. On this particular ward of this particular hospital, at least.

OK, it's better than the last place. I have a separate room, containing a small bed with plastic sheeting underneath and a rubber pillow. There is a sink and a wardrobe with a door that is wedged half open.

The ward is built alongside a railway line. I sit on the bed and stare out of the window at the yellowing sycamore leaves. Tube trains rattle past till 1am then start again around 5. A light flickers overhead. Staff peek in all night long. They don't make huge efforts to be quiet.

It really isn't conducive to sleep, which, if anyone remembers that far back, is the reason I'm in this bloody mess in the first place.

Therapy is almost non-existent, except for an 'art room' with three crayons and some plasticine. Sorry, I'm just not going there: I still have a tiny shred of self-respect. Interestingly, there is one group session where a psychologist comes along and we discuss Maslow's Hierarchy of Needs – a pyramid-shaped diagram of what humans require, from food and sex, to 'self-actualization'. The session is surprisingly intellectual and I rally a bit.

Otherwise, there isn't much to do. The TV is on without sound all day.

I discover half of a Frank Sinatra biography (the second half). At least I know how the story ends. (Never lovers, ever friends.)

Three times a day, a bossy nurse marches down the corridors shouting, 'Fresh air! Fresh air!' Everyone dutifully shuffles out to a courtyard so small, surrounded by such high walls that you can barely see the sky. I had a day trip to Benidorm once; it reminds me of that.

The yard resembles a large ashtray. It *stinks* of tobacco. I am the only patient who isn't smoking. The air is actually fresher on the ward.

I don't want my family to visit me here. But Anthony, my former therapist, arrives with the most enormous bar of chocolate.

14th November

0 HOURS, 0 MINUTES

The nursing staff treat patients as an irritation. You actually see their eyes glazing over when you ask for help. They are more like jailers, really – and I guess they have to be because most patients here are 'sectioned', or held under the Mental Health Act. The nurses are all tall and they look straight over my head into the middle distance as I plead for assistance.

I am a voluntary patient but, even so, the nurses don't want to let me out, even for a walk in the hospital grounds. This upsets me greatly. Unlike most of the patients, I haven't been sectioned and should be free to come and go as I please.

The nurses are only there for crowd-control and to dispense meds, it seems. They are not compassionate.

The only person who is kind to me is a student mental health nurse who looks barely 19. She can't do anything but at least she listens.

15th November

0 HOURS, 0 MINUTES

During this stay I only recall seeing a doctor once.

Memories are hazy but the young consultant decides to keep my medications as they are. This is disappointing, as part of my warped logic for checking in was to try a new approach.

He suggests I try to get a job: 'Maybe in Tesco?'

16th November

0 HOURS, 0 MINUTES

A male patient comes into the women's side and poos in the bath. We all move into the men's side for a few hours while it's cleaned up.

17th November

0 HOURS, 0 MINUTES

I try to speak to some of the patients, but – as you would imagine – many of them are very ill. (As am I, of course.) Conversations start off reasonably, then people start sharing their plans for world domination. One man takes out his book of indecipherable rantings about railway lines and how they are the key to 'the universe' and there I am stuck for an hour and a half.

Two people stand out for me: a former table-football champion (we played on the ward table – I scored a goal! I think she was heavily medicated!) and a sweet, younger boy who wears a Manchester United kit every day. We watch a Champions League match together.

Most of the rest of the time, this tiny boy is being man-handled into a scary looking padded room and injected into the bottom while several large nurses hold him down.

Manchester United win their match, thank goodness.

18th November

0 HOURS, 0 MINUTES

After five days or so, there is a 'ward round', where the young consultant and a bunch of other people I don't recognize discuss my case, while I look silently on.

I am deemed something of a time-waster and am immediately kicked out, back to the ministrations of the Home Treatment Team.

20th November

0 HOURS, 0 MINUTES

I make a resolution. I am going to come off all my drugs.

The whole point of starting medication was to sleep. But it's a shit sandwich. I'm still not sleeping and I'm still addicted to the pills.

Rehab was a disaster. The NHS is hopeless. *The Ashton Manual* requires self-discipline (and maths skills) that I do not possess.

So, I am going to do it by myself.

I'm not quite stupid enough to go 'cold turkey' – I know that could be fatal. And as I have already cut down from 50mg to 20mg of Valium, some of the heavy lifting has been done already. Online research tells me that trazodone, my anti-depressant, doesn't have any withdrawal effects, or only minor ones.

So, I decide on my own taper. I can't be arsed to write out a reduction programme. It's rather haphazard.

But you know what? After everything I've been through, how could things possibly be worse?

I'll be abstinent and clean, like the 12 Steps require. I will eat kale. Drink lots of water. Say affirmations. Maybe even take up yoga.

Then, surely, my unsullied brain will tell itself: 'Oh yes. *That's* what you need to sleep again.' And reboot.

25th December

O HOURS, O MINUTES

Christmas passes in a haze. I am mostly up in my bedroom, Googling new physical symptoms. My family make a meal. I bolt it down and rush back up to the safety of my bedroom where I concentrate on not taking as many pills.

Year Five

9th January

0 HOURS, 0 MINUTES

By now, I am off all the drugs except for a small dose of Valium. Things really are blurry now. I can't recall how much I am on. My family are going away for the weekend.

I decide that – with no one else in the house – this represents a good opportunity to 'jump off' altogether. Stop taking everything. Get it over with.

I take my last Valium on Friday afternoon. I can feel myself becoming increasingly jittery by Saturday lunchtime, so I put on *This Is Us,* the One Direction movie. I'm sure Harry, Zayn and co. can shepherd me through this.

Things progress. The shaking and sweating I have done before. And the nausea. But even I am unprepared for the stabbing-in-the-guts-curl-up-in-a-ball-on-the-floor mental torture that overwhelms me by the time the final credits roll.

I am rolling around, clutching my sides. Moaning so loud, I'm sure the neighbours can hear me.

Then my memory goes very hazy.

But I do recall a new, weird thing starts to emerge. I start hitting myself in the face. A bit like Dustin Hoffman in *Rain Man*.

Nope. I have no idea why, either.

Year Ten: A note from the future

Professor Joanna Moncrieff, author of *A Straight Talking Introduction to Psychiatric Drugs*, has this to say:

'Abrupt cessation of benzodiazepines can lead to psychotic symptoms, confusion, suicidal impulses and other behavioural disturbances that were not present before the drug was started.

'Withdrawal reactions usually start within hours or days of stopping or reducing the dose, depending on the half life of the drug. For long-acting benzodiazepines such as diazepam (Valium), withdrawal reactions can be delayed, sometimes by a few weeks.

'Latest estimates suggest that everyone who takes benzodiazepines for a period of six months or more will show some degree of withdrawal following discontinuation of the drugs. It has been known since the 1980s that withdrawal symptoms can often last for many months.

'They may wax and wane in severity and usually they improve gradually over time. However, some people continue to have severe or protracted withdrawal symptoms that can last for months or years. Sometimes, these protracted withdrawal symptoms can mimic common disorders like depression. Symptoms can be so severe and debilitating that people are unable to get off the drugs, even though they want to.

'If they push through and do not return to medication, they may have to endure significantly reduced quality of life for months, or even years, afterwards.

'There is a serious lack of research on how to withdraw safely and effectively from psychiatric drugs. In many cases, we do not have information about exactly how fast or slowly withdrawal should be conducted. There are some situations in which sudden withdrawal can be life-threatening. As with alcohol, rapid withdrawal from high-dose benzodiazepines can cause epileptic fits and severe withdrawal reactions, for example.

'In these circumstances, it is important that withdrawal is carried out slowly and carefully, with medical supervision.'

13th January

O HOURS, O MINUTES

My wider family have become involved. Today, they have made me an appointment with a consultant based at a private psychiatric clinic.

All I recall about this session is the swirly pattern on the hall carpet on the way to the doctor's office. Then being led to a bedroom which is certainly a step above the NHS facilities, though not the luxury that people imagine these celebrity haunts to have. It's more like a three-star hotel.

So I have been admitted to the clinic. It's very expensive and so my father has offered to pay.

14th January

O HOURS, O MINUTES

Before I try to shore the fragments against my ruins of this particular stay, I'm going to type out excerpts of the psychiatrist's letter that accompanied me on my discharge.

This'll give you an idea of how a medical expert saw me at the time.

'When Miranda was admitted under my care, her mental state was as such that she presented with a severe presentation of depression, alongside delusional beliefs that her body was being destroyed. She reported having been living in the loft conversion of her house separate from the rest of her family. She described having social, family and economical problems. Her mental state was not good and she had been under the care of the NHS for many years.

'Miranda presented with psychotic symptoms from the beginning of the admission and was therefore put on, initially, olanzapine* 2.5mg up to 20mg daily and Fluanxol** 1mg daily. Due to the depressive symptoms she was

---

* An anti-psychotic drug, which famously has weight gain as a side effect.
** A drug, I have just discovered, that is used for schizophrenia. *Schizophrenia*?

also started on venlafaxine XL* 75mg. Her mental state improved steadily. She was able to attend groups on her last day of admission and also socialize and eat in the dining room with other patients.

'At the beginning of the admission she was withdrawing from any social interaction and slapped her face continuously.

'Two days before discharge, Miranda requested to change olanzapine to another anti-psychotic medication because she felt she was putting weight on too rapidly. She was concerned about the way she looked, which indicated that she was more caring about herself. Olanzapine 20mg was changed to risperidone** 3mg and she was discharged taking risperidone 3mg and venlafaxine XL 75mg.'

The definition of psychosis

Psychosis is when people lose some contact with reality. This might involve seeing or hearing things that other people cannot see or hear (hallucinations) and believing things that are not actually true (delusions).

The two main symptoms of psychosis are:

Hallucinations: Where a person hears, sees and, in some cases, feels, smells or tastes things that do not exist outside their mind but nonetheless feel very real to them. Hearing voices is a common hallucination.

---

* An SNRI anti-depressant (see page 47).
** An older anti-psychotic that's not meant to be as associated with weight gain.

Delusions: Where a person has strong beliefs that are not shared by others. A common delusion is someone believing there's a conspiracy to harm them.

I certainly never hallucinated or heard voices. As for the delusions, well, I know for a fact this psychiatrist thought my non-sleep was a delusion. He also humoured me when I complained about my physical indignities.

His letter basically says I am mad, a diagnosis I do not dispute at all. It is not normal for a person to sit in their bed 24 hours a day, slapping their face.

Psychiatrist Dr Sami Timimi on psychosis

'For over 100 years, there has been a basic difference in psychiatry between a "neurotic illness", where you are thought to remain in touch with reality, and a "psychotic" one, where you have lost touch with reality. This definition has a long and troubling history. The best-known psychotic illness is schizophrenia.

'Three main things define psychosis: a thought disorder, delusions and hallucinations (or abnormal perceptions). In the *Diagnostic and Statistical Manual* (the mental health diagnosis manual), you are diagnosed with a psychotic illness if you tick a certain number of boxes.

'From the letter above, and from what you have told me – and if you believe the system is valid – you probably did reach the criteria for psychotic depression. But it's a subjective system. There were understandable reasons that you presented like that. I have seen all sorts of unusual symptoms from patients suffering with sleep deprivation.

'Olanzapine and risperidone are "dirty drugs". They block a number of brain chemicals, but mostly dopamine, which can then turn a patient into a zombie, rather than putting them to sleep, and stop a person feeling enjoyment. Blocking dopamine causes a Parkinsonian-like state, a numbness. Anti-psychotics also mess up your metabolic system, interfering with insulin sensitivity and growth hormones. I'm not at all surprised you put on weight.

'There is also a rare syndrome called akathisia – a movement disorder characterized by a feeling of inner restlessness, accompanied by mental distress and an inability to sit still.

'I do think there is a place for anti-psychotic drugs but probably in fewer than about 5 per cent of cases where they are currently prescribed. If a person is in a highly aroused state of mind, has lost touch with reality and is a risk to themselves or someone else, these medications can reduce the levels of emotional intensity, so we can start a conversation.

'As a physician, I would only prescribe anti-psychotics in these acute situations, on a low dose, and aim to bring the patient off them as soon as possible.'

15th January

0 HOURS, 0 MINUTES

I do tell the psychiatrist – on more than one occasion – that I have just come off benzodiazepines rather quickly after being on a high dose for almost five years. The doctor does not think this is an issue, waves it aside – and moves swiftly on.

My insomnia is dismissed early on in favour of a diagnosis which sounds something like a 'dopamine deficiency' – the sort of term one might use to placate a patient who doesn't understand anything about psychiatry.

I am so loopy-loo that I cannot sufficiently bang the drum about the effect of my lack of sleep and my concern about the benzo withdrawals. Nowhere in my diagnosis or treatment plan is either of these taken into account, nor are they to be referenced in the longer version of my discharge letter.

I feel this is significant.

1st February

O HOURS, O MINUTES

I was agoraphobic before my admission into this hospital. Since returning from rehab, I had stopped going outside at all. Yet at least I moved from room to room within my house.

But here I don't even want to leave my bedroom. Despite the constant encouragements of staff, I refuse to mingle with the other patients or attend the therapy groups (unlike at the NHS hospital, there is a full programme of therapy). Nor do I want to go to the dining room.

I can't even face the walk down the hall to visit the consultant, who has an office on site.

There is a rule that I have to be 'checked on' every 15 minutes in case, I guess, I try to hang myself from the plastic curtain rail or the doorknob that is round and slippery so you can't hang yourself from it.

Because it's a private hospital and I am a paying customer, the staff are initially content to bring meals to my room. As my stay continues, however, they understandably become less happy to do so. The windows in the rooms only open a fraction – to prevent escapes, presumably – and my room starts to smell.

All I do is stare at the newspaper, gaze at the TV, slap my face and babble that I can't sleep. And I eat. There are three cooked meals a day (including breakfast) plus stodgy puddings and custard with lunch and dinner. I constantly crave carbohydrates. Once, I make a rare foray into the kitchen to make a cup of tea, spot someone's left-over treacle pudding and eat it.

No one has a bloody clue what to do with me.

I can't remember the last time I wore make-up or had a haircut. I often wear the same set of clothes two or three days in a row. I think my appearance is staring to alarm people. (Is this paranoid? Not sure.)

The staff on the 15-minute rota have a habit of walking into the room and then knocking afterwards, rather than the other way around. You can't lock your door, for safety reasons. A 'health assistant' barges in on me while I am in the bath. I hear sniggers and unkind whisperings in the hallway outside. Or maybe that's also my paranoia.

It doesn't occur to me (or anyone else, for that matter) that my nutty behaviour might be down to my over-rapid benzo withdrawals.

19th February

0 HOURS, 0 MINUTES

Hamlet said: 'I could be bounded in a nutshell, and count myself a king of infinite space, were it not that I have bad dreams.' I hear him. I am also cabin'd, cribb'd, confined.

Hamlet also said: 'To die, to sleep – to sleep, perchance to dream.' Lucky bugger. The Danish prince had it rough but even *he* got some sleep at night.

3rd March

0 HOURS, 0 MINUTES

The consultant's discharge letter concludes thus:

'There were a lot of discussions regarding continuation of care [...] Miranda was discharged to her own home in a relatively better mental state than she was before. The worry is that Miranda lacks insight in regard to her delusional beliefs, and that she would stop taking the medication.

'Therefore, on discharge, a private mental health coach was hired to visit Miranda at her home.'

10th March

0 HOURS, 0 MINUTES

The private mental health coach, C, comes to my house. C is well-meaning with a no-nonsense air. But all she really achieves in the fortnight or so that she visits is to rootle through my wardrobe in a women's magaziney 'declutter your life' sort of a way and throw out my £2,000 wedding dress. 'We won't be needing that anymore,' she says, as I watch aghast. Plans I may have had to hand this beautiful gown to my daughter are immediately thwarted.

However, I do manage to dive across and hurl myself on top of the £400 Fenwick's leather jacket which was also destined for the recycling. A primeval instinct has emerged in which I vaguely imagine a future where I might wear such a thing again.

Is this a glimmer of recovery?

C even takes me on a trip to the local shopping mall. I find this place hell in normal times, so you can imagine how it feels today, especially when I see my swelling arse in one of those 'show you the back' mirrors.

Ultimately, it's about more than new clothes and I'm afraid C's ministrations don't really help. She doesn't come cheap, either, and we part company after two weeks.

I know I am not an easy person to help. Everyone who tries tells me so.

25th March

0 HOURS, 0 MINUTES

If there was a spark of recovery when I came out of hospital, it is soon extinguished.

I have been ridiculed in rehab, thrown out of an NHS psychiatric hospital and spent several tens of thousands of pounds of my father's money in a private clinic where pills for the long-term mad have been thrown at me. Even the wonderful Anthony refers to me as a 'basket case'. (He says it in an affectionate tone but I take everything at face value these days and am a humour-free zone.)

People on the whole used to like me. I mean not everyone, obviously – and I could be tough and outspoken in my editor's capacity – but in general, new acquaintances would smile, engage and at least pretend to tolerate me. Now I feel an immediate recoil in the air, from everyone from doctors to clinic receptionists to my friends who barely visit anymore (largely because I don't want them to, it's so awful for everyone).

In fact, the only people I ever really see these days are my immediate family and mental health professionals.

'Healthy Miranda' is not generally given to self-pity. But I am not really 'Miranda' anymore.

Which leads me to thinking: what is 'Miranda'? What makes a person 'a person'? How is their identity built? Is it their job? Their place in the family hierarchy? Their friends? Recognizing their reflection in the mirror and quietly approving of it? A mixture of the above?

I remember briefly questioning my identity once before. Like many women, I found early maternity leave a challenge, being stuck at home with mewling and puking babies – two born within twenty months of one another – away from the fun and independence of my career. I was never diagnosed with postnatal depression and I don't think I had it. But I do remember feeling flat and bored for a lot of the early days. And above all, exhausted. For the first six months, those breastfed terrors rarely slept for more than an hour at a time before they woke up demanding a meal. And then another one.

Yes, I was drained with sleeplessness and more than once wanted to hurl said babies out of the window like a rugby ball. But it was different from the tortures of my Insomnia Crash. The minute the babies dropped off, I did, too.

Sleep was waiting for me, it just needed an opportunity. Now, I have plenty of opportunity – 24 hours of it! – but no sleep.

When they were six weeks old, my babies started to smile. My lost, hopeless feeling started to lift and when I resumed my work and socializing, my identity came rushing back. The unresponsive newborns grew up and became fascinating little people.

This current state, however, feels permanent. There is no job to go back to. I have lost my more peripheral friends. If you saw a photo of me five years ago, you would not believe it was the same person. There is no light at the end of the tunnel.

I am so depleted, crushed, despairing that I don't have the energy to even think about suicide any longer.

25th April

O HOURS, O MINUTES

At some point I go for a 'medical review' with a psychiatrist, a new one. Maybe there is more than one – I don't remember. From the haze I do recall that the anti-psychotics are substituted with different ones, then stopped altogether. Someone puts me on zopiclone, the sleeping pill that doesn't appear to work. A sedative anti-depressant called mirtazapine is added in. My Psychiatric Safari continues.

It's a mess. I am a guinea pig in a psychiatry lab. But do you know what? I don't give a shit anymore. I've given up trying to control any of this.

Pills, water, swallow. Repeat.

What I do all day: Stare at the TV, make huge rounds of toast, eat multipacks of crisps. If there is a bottle of wine downstairs, I will drink it. This is a new thing.

I am putting on weight in a very strange way. My arms and legs are still skinny, but my stomach is protruding. A bit like a spider.

For some reason, I have become very interested in football and watch repeats of *Match of the Day* on my laptop. Football is kind of like a soap opera and I become invested, tuning into talkSPORT for the latest goss. The biggest event of the year is when José Mourinho gets sacked from Chelsea for the second time.

I read footballer Zlatan Ibrahimović's wild biography – he's a riot! – on a Kindle kindly donated by my cousin. Then, in my usual balanced way, I go back and start it again, and reread my favourite bits. (It was good, but not *that* good.)

My vision has started deteriorating – hence the Kindle, which is easier to read. It's got so bad that I can barely see out of one eye. Might this have something to do with the episodes where I hit myself in the face? 'I can't seeeeee,' is added to 'I can't sleeeeeep.'

Once or twice, I have a spike of desperation, which leads to a panic attack where I struggle to breathe. I call an ambulance and expect a day trip to A&E. The first time, I am driven to the hospital and – vital stats taken and found to be normal – I am immediately wheeled out the back door again. The second time I call 999, the paramedics sit in my front room, make sure my oxygen levels are OK, then leave without taking me anywhere.

What I do all night: Read Zlatan's biography, listen to talkSPORT, eat toast, will the morning not to come. I have started writing a saga of epic novels in my head – racy and convoluted. The characters have children – and then grandchildren. It's quite intriguing. I don't write a word down but this is an imaginary world into which I can escape.

This state of affairs will continue for the rest of the year and into the following one.

What I don't do is sleep.

Year Six

15th July

O HOURS, O MINUTES

Let's put aside the trivial issue of my sanity for a moment. My eyesight has got really bad and I am almost completely blind in one eye.

My father has just retired from his dental practice and thus has more time to help me. He books me an appointment with a private eye surgeon near his home.

The surgeon takes one look at me and says it's an emergency. I have a detached retina that needs to be operated on without delay. I also have cataracts that will need removing at a later date. I am 48.

6th August

2 HOURS, 30 MINUTES UNDER A GENERAL ANAESTHETIC (BUT THAT REALLY DOESN'T COUNT, DOES IT?)

I am being prepped for a general anaesthetic. I am, of course, worried about my sight but more concerned that the anaesthetic won't work – I'm convinced that insomnia extends also to industrial-strength sedatives. I've been through enough and don't really need to be awake while a surgeon slices through my eye with a scalpel, thank you very much.

But I needn't have worried. I'm knocked out flat, without even that cosy little countdown you see them doing in the movies. When I come around, resplendent in an eyepatch, I vomit all over the auxiliary nurse. 'I didn't sign up for this,' she mutters.

I had hoped that being 'out' for a couple of hours might feel a bit like sleep and maybe a bit refreshing.

It really isn't. I feel even more dreadful than usual. But, when I lift up the eyepatch to take a peek at the world, I can see again.

7th August

0 HOURS, 0 MINUTES

It is decided that I will recuperate at my father's home, especially as I have some further (less invasive) surgery coming up. I arrive with only an overnight bag but will be hanging around in PJs, so what else could I possibly need?

8th–21st August

0 HOURS, 0 MINUTES

The Olympic games. I watch every second of it, from the early morning kayaking, to the diving and the dressage. I even show up for the medal ceremonies.

29th August

O HOURS, O MINUTES

Arguably the lowest point in this whole shebang. The only pair of shoes I have with me are the old downtrodden Uggs in which I arrived.

My dad takes me to Sports Direct, where he chooses for me a pair of white trainers with pink trim, *that do up with Velcro straps.*

7th September

O HOURS, O MINUTES

Four weeks later and I am still at my father's house.* The great news is that my eyesight has been saved, though subsequent cataract operations will change my vision to permanent long-sightedness. I will need to wear glasses for the rest of my life.

Eye operations are not fun, nor is being dependent on spectacles, but to be able to see is rather nice. I don't appreciate that to the full right now but, in the future, I most certainly will.

No explicit conversation takes place but it transpires I am going to stay at my dad's. This decision is best for everyone: myself, my ex and especially my kids. I have been MIA Mummy for far too long, now.

---

* By the way, thanks Dad. I don't like the loose use of the word 'literally', but it's appropriate here. You may have quite literally saved my life by opening up your home to me.

We agree that Dad will look after my tablets so I am not tempted to take more than I should. He leaves them out at 6pm every evening in a blue egg cup that says 'Flamborough' on it. This makes me feel even more like a child. If going to live with my father in middle age had not finished that job already.

The care coordinator drives over to formally sign me off her watch. She wishes me well and even gives me a hug. But I'm sure I hear her skipping as she crunches off down the gravel.

I am now without a psychiatrist. Maybe that's not such a bad thing for a while.

28th September

0 HOURS, 0 MINUTES

I've been at my dad's place for nearly two months now. I had hoped that in a new environment, I might be feeling better and even sleeping a little.

But this is not the case.

I am no longer hitting myself, on pain of death from my eye surgeon who says I really *will* go blind. But nothing else has really changed that much. I still sit in my bed – just a different one. My dad has a cupboard full of Scottish butter shortbread and I make frequent trips to said cupboard.

My friends live an hour's drive away. I left my (analogue, pay-as-you-go) mobile at the house and it gets thrown away. So even if I wanted to contact people, I don't have their details.

Not that this means much to me, anymore.

5th October

47 MINUTES – SCATTERED WILLY-NILLY – SAYS THE SLEEP TRACKER. BUT SORRY, I JUST DON'T BUY IT

My dad buys me a sleep tracker. I try this huge chunk of black plastic for three nights in a row. Not only does it not help me to sleep, it's bloody uncomfortable.

When I examine the statistics the next morning, they tell me I slept a few minutes here and there, but these were at times I knew I was actually downstairs or having a bath.

On the third evening, I take the sleep tracker off and throw it at the wall.

On sleep trackers

At some point during my Insomnia Crash, the world went mad for sleep trackers.

But many experts are sceptical of these devices. They argue that they might even be harming our sleep, that the obsession with how long we sleep, and how well, does us no good at all.

There's even a flashy, scientific-sounding name for this syndrome: 'orthosomnia'.

The phrase originated in a 2017 report in the *Journal of Clinical Sleep Medicine*, after an American neurologist and her colleagues noticed 'a perfectionist quest to achieve perfect sleep'. The word orthosomnia mirrors that of orthorexia, which has been used for the past 20 years as a buzzword for obsessively healthy eating.

Much of this preoccupation comes from the rise of the sleep tracker family. Doctors noted that people were stressed out – and, in some cases, their sleep was suffering further – because they weren't measuring up to their tracker's definition of 'good' sleep and felt disappointed. As well as baffled and obsessed with new terminology, such as sleep debt percentages, heart rate dips, graphs of sleep disruptions and comparisons to other users.

Professor Guy Leschziner is a consultant neurologist who runs the Sleep Disorders Centre at Guy's Hospital in London. He is also the author of *The Nocturnal Brain: Nightmares, Neuroscience and the Secret World of Sleep*.

'Several years ago, we started noticing that patients were turning up to their appointments with sleep trackers, which they used to report how much sleep they'd had the night before,' he says. 'We weren't entirely surprised, because of the developments in devices that counted people's steps, or how many calories they had consumed that day.'

Leschziner agrees with the American researchers' concerns that the pursuit of bedtime perfection can be a problem.

'For starters, sleep trackers are not accurate,' he says. 'Yes, they can monitor the time you have spent in bed, based on your movement. Some of the more sophisticated can tell you how long you have been asleep. But what they cannot do is tell the quality of sleep; what stage of sleep you are at at a certain time or how many times you have woken up during the night.'

And this is bad because? 'Anything that draws attention to sleep can make it worse,' says Professor Leschziner. 'This is why people fall asleep while watching TV or reading a book. They are distracted. But if you feel you have poor-quality sleep, and the tracker confirms this, it won't help but will only increase your anxiety.'

The original orthosomnia researchers agreed. They found that patients had been spending more time in bed to improve their 'sleep numbers', which may have made their insomnia worse.

And so far we've been talking about people who sleep reasonably well. But what about those – like me – who already suffer with chronic insomnia? Surely sticking a plastic 'watch' on them is bad enough. But then to have their worse suspicions confirmed, or perhaps distorted, because of inaccurate data?

So should you bin the sleep tracker? 'If a device like this can help make positive lifestyle changes in diet and exercise, then it can't be a bad thing,' says Professor Leschziner. 'But sleep trackers do not contribute to the treatment of insomnia. In fact, they may do significant harm.'

5th December

O HOURS, O MINUTES

I discover my father's iPad and streaming services.

My obsession moves to movies. I devour entire film genres: World War Two movies, everything Michael Fassbender and Ryan Gosling have ever appeared in, the Marvel superhero films, documentaries about the Beatles. You have to pay for many of these, so I just click away, adding to the account which is billed to my father.

Dad moans constantly at me to cut down on my spending. But perhaps he is secretly pleased that I am looking outside myself a bit. Maybe it is a good thing.

Other than this, I eat and eat. I take pills. That's all really.

Since moving home, I have been without a psychiatrist, just continuing on a repeat prescription. Before Christmas, we decide that I should probably sign up to the care of a professional.

There is a wait of six weeks or so, then I find myself in a familiar scenario – albeit in a different office, with a new consultant.

Year Seven

23rd January

0 HOURS, 0 MINUTES

I go to see Dr D. I ramble out the same old tale of woe. He writes to my GP.

Three things I like about this letter:

- There is reference to my benzodiazepine dependency and an explicit note that I have never – before or since – had a problem with alcohol or drugs.
- That my 'premorbid' personality is taken into account: I was 'well above average' in my education, succeeded in my career and had a series of successful relationships. I am a person, not just a collection of labels, diagnoses and pills.
- The doctor concludes I don't have – and never have had – a personality disorder and am instead suffering with recurrent depressive disorder.

Two things I don't like about this letter:

- This paragraph: 'Miranda tells me she has not slept for years. This is obviously unbelievable but is unfortunately how Miranda feels at the moment. With this in mind, my intention is to undertake a detailed review of her medication.'

- Suggested in this medication review: I am to reduce mirtazapine (apparently, I have been on a whacking dose) and put back on trazadone. I'm to start taking pregabalin again. Pregabalin is the anti-seizure medication that is prescribed 'off label' for anxiety.

My doctor tells me it has no side effects or withdrawal symptoms. I'm to stay on zopiclone, the sleeping pill that hasn't worked thus far. Fair enough. To come off that seems a bit perverse.

Dr D also recommends I start taking lithium, a 'mood stabilizer' which was an old-fashioned treatment for bipolar disorder, or manic depression. He says it might make my anti-depressants work better.

What he skates over is this: lithium can cause tremors and problems with kidney function. He plays this down but can't quite answer my repeated questions about why patients on lithium need regular blood tests.

I do not wish to take it and gracefully decline.

Says Dr Sami Timimi from the future: 'Thank God you didn't take lithium. It's toxic.'

3rd February

0 HOURS, 0 MINUTES

'Tis the season of Nexflix 'n' pills, and the biscuit cupboard.

Not much changes. I am still sleepless. And though I'm not actively doing loopy-loo things like slapping myself in the face, I am still not capable of a conversation beyond the usual 'I can't sleep'. My words come out in a repetitive stutter. I am still agoraphobic, socially phobic and generally useless to mankind.

On the other hand, I am venturing downstairs more. I occasionally even go out into the garden at 6am for some early morning sun.

And what do I do all day?

BOX SETS!

So, yes, Amazon Video and Netflix. I sign up and an Aladdin's cave opens in front of me. Endless exciting TV shows with 'seasons' that go on for *ever*. They include:

- *Mad Men* (advertising in the sixties! Secretaries! Cocktails!)
- *Breaking Bad* (I devour the epic of Walter White in *two* weeks – that's something)
- *The Americans* (underrated, and brilliant)
- *Fauda, Srugim* and *Shtisel* (I adore these Israeli shows, especially all the eating and the smoking in *Shtisel*)
- *Broadchurch* and *The Night Manager* (which set me off looking for everything Tom Hiddleston has ever done, especially featuring his bottom)

This lot keeps me busy for a while.

15th June

O HOURS, O MINUTES

Dr D has left the NHS to go private because he's annoyed about their restructuring programme. (I suspect his bank balance may have something to do with it.) I am now face-to-face with Dr F.

Dr F is cheerful, he listens, is persuasive and tries again to put me on lithium.

According to my medical notes, it seems that I agreed at the time – but the minute I leave his office, I change my mind.

Year Eight

1st March

O HOURS, O MINUTES

My new health authority sends around G, a mental health worker, who is to visit me every week for a defined period. G is open-minded and sweet. But we don't get off to the best of starts.

The very first thing she says on hearing my story is: 'Well, maybe you should accept you are never going to sleep again and just get on with your life.'

And, as for my insistence that I haven't slept for eight years and that no one believes me: 'Well, would *you* believe you?'

This does not initially endear her to me.

6th June

O HOURS, O MINUTES

Dr F again. He notes thus: 'Miranda has no periods of respite: she continues to experience generalized feelings of anxiety on a daily basis.'

He says, 'There is no evidence of psychotic symptoms.' Then, Dr F goes on to prescribe me 7.5mg olanzapine, which is an anti-psychotic. Go figure.

I am also put on a waiting list for 'talking' therapy, via something called IAPT (Improving Access to Psychological Therapies) a newish NHS initiative which aims to move away from drug prescribing. Which can only be a good thing.

7th June

O HOURS, O MINUTES

Why do I start taking the olanzapine again?

Well, I'm clearly still not right. And when I say 'no' yet again to the lithium deal, Dr F looks a bit put out. There aren't many choices left, he says. We will have come to the end of the psychiatric road.

I don't want to be sacked by my consultant. But nor do I want to be a shaking wreck with buggered-up kidneys, so I choose the pills that make you fat, instead, and take one for the team.

29th June

O HOURS, O MINUTES

I wonder why olanzapine makes you fat while tearing open a pack of Jaffa Cakes. I take two of them from the pack and stomp my way upstairs.

Then I fancy a couple more. 'Oh, I don't give a fuck,' I tell myself. 'Might as well finish the lot.'

I constantly crave carbohydrates and never seem to get full. Cereal bars, oven chip wedges, Ambrosia rice pudding. Toast at 3am 'doesn't count', I say. I never weigh myself.

15th July

O HOURS, O MINUTES

I'm still a total mess but G the mental health worker is making me *do* things.

I don't want to do them, I want to sit in bed and watch another episode of *Outlander*, but G and my father conspire to bully that these things are 'good for me'. So I reluctantly comply.

G and I go for walk-and-talks around the block. These are more like stumble-and-pantings. I am totally unfit and have to stop for breath several times, even on a single circuit.

But . . . I do talk. For the first time in years.

I recount with bittersweet nostalgia my days in journalism: the excitement of filing an article at 7pm and seeing it in the newspaper at 5am the next day. Or the fun of being a magazine editor 'auditioning' babies for cover shoots.

The nostalgia is more bitter than sweet because it's clear to me that part of my life is over.

I remember how the counsellors in rehab said that 'euphoric recall' around booze and drugs is a bad thing. Well, this is my version of euphoric recall.

'Don't dwell on all that,' G says. 'You need to find a new life, now. Make some new friends. Perhaps a part-time job in an office?'

But I *liked* my old career. I *liked* my old friends. *I loved my life.*

8th August

O HOURS, O MINUTES

G also has a habit of dragging me out to a coffee shop in the local town, an expedition I loathe. I insist we sit in a corner, where no one can see me – I am that self-conscious about the way I look.

G asks me what I want to drink. I look blank, then I say: 'Well, the Old Miranda would have liked Earl Grey tea.'

G beams. 'No, this is what *Miranda* likes. That's great! We need to find that part of you again.'

It sounds so minor but actually, she might be right. Maybe it's too grand a plan to think about becoming a journalist again. But in the same way I rediscovered my identity after becoming a mother, maybe I need to start taking baby steps. With hot beverages.

G orders the Earl Grey while I scuttle off to find a dark, corner table. Despite my continuing general misery, I enjoy my tea. We might have hit on something here.

What else did Old Miranda like, that can be imported to a New Miranda?

31st August

0 HOURS, 0 MINUTES

Last week, a letter came through, telling me I have moved up the therapy waiting list. I can start a six-week NHS course this week.

You know I am not really a 'group-y' person. Rehab made me hate 'groups' even more. And my preoccupation with how terrible I look *really* makes me not want to go. But G and Dr F are doing their best for me, so I have to show willing at least. Who knows? Maybe the answer is there.

The course is billed as 'CBT for Anxiety'. While I argue – and still do, some years on – that anxiety was never a problem for me in my 'premorbid' life, it clearly is right now.

I know I am fat. I see that my hair and skin look terrible. None of these things stop a mentally healthy person from leaving the house. On the rare occasion I speak to friends, they tell me to 'stop being so vain'.

Anyway, the group is today. I pack a notebook and something to write with, prise open my mind and go to the first anxiety session.

We participants are a right old real raggle-taggle across the mental health spectrum. Some people are clearly quite unwell. Others have taken afternoons off work and I can't see anything wrong with them.

The facilitator circulates handout on top of handout about the causes of anxiety and a simple explanation of the theory behind CBT. There is a whiteboard with coloured marker pens. The facilitator writes the word 'fear' on the whiteboard and asks us to come up with synonyms for it.

We spend an hour discussing the meaning of 'fear'.
Then we are out of time.

7th September

O HOURS, O MINUTES

Part two of the CBT for Anxiety course. We all go round
and say how we are doing.

One middle-aged man starts to talk about his carpen-
try, the boat he is building and the performance of one
of his lathes. He goes on and on, uninterrupted for 20
minutes. He's clearly not entirely with the programme. In
fact, his discourse gets quite aggressive at times and it's
disconcerting.

I gaze out of the window and dream of Donald Draper.

Not only does this course feel like a waste of time, it's
actually upsetting me. I resolve to pack it in.

10th September

O HOURS, O MINUTES

But still, I don't sleep.

From the frazzled neurons of my brain comes a thought.
I've had insomnia for almost a decade now. There *has* to be
a more effective treatment than drugs and the entry-level
talking therapy offered by the NHS.

Maybe things have moved on since I first sought treatment.

Last week, I begged my father to help me find another way. He has heard of a private GP with a sympathetic reputation. Tonight, the doctor comes to call.

The GP tells me there is an NHS 'sleep clinic' based within a 90-minute drive. I am ecstatic. How come this has never shown up in my Googling before? The doctor promises to write a referral letter to the clinic. 'We offer diagnostic tests and treatments to people with a great range of sleep disorders from all around the UK,' reads its impressive website. This bodes well!

17th October

0 HOURS, 0 MINUTES

Five weeks after seeing the private GP, I rock up at the sleep clinic. The waiting room is full of large people trailing contraptions on wheels. I soon discover these are 'CPAP' machines, which pump air through a mask that people with a breathing condition called sleep apnoea wear at night.

I have some health checks: blood pressure, Body Mass Index. Then I see a delightful Polish doctor who is the only medical professional to believe that I have not slept for eight years. I want to hug him.

The doctor agrees to admit me for overnight tests – tests which will tell me how much I sleep, if at all. From the results, we will see what we can do about it. I feel optimistic.

The anatomy of sleep

Sleep involves several areas of the brain:

- The hypothalamus, a peanut-sized structure deep inside the brain, contains groups of nerve cells that act as control centres affecting sleep and arousal. Inside the hypothalamus is the suprachiasmatic nucleus (SCN) – a cluster of thousands of cells that receive information about light exposure directly from your eyes and control your circadian rhythm. Even blind people maintain some ability to sense light and are able to modify their sleep–wake cycle.

- The brain stem communicates with the hypothalamus to control the transitions between wake and sleep. Sleep-promoting cells within the hypothalamus and the brain stem produce a brain chemical called GABA, which reduces the arousal of your hypothalamus and the brain stem. The brain stem also plays a special role in REM sleep (see opposite), sending signals for your muscles to relax. This is essential for body posture and limb movements, so that you don't start rushing about during nightmares.

- The thalamus relays information to the cerebral cortex (the covering of the brain that interprets and processes information from short- to long-term memory). During most stages of sleep, the thalamus calms down, so you can tune out the external world. But during REM sleep, the thalamus is active, sending the cortex images, sounds and other sensations that fill our dreams.

- The pineal gland receives signals from the SCN and increases production of the hormone melatonin

(see page 32), which knocks you out as it gets dark.
Scientists believe that peaks and valleys of melatonin
over time are important for matching the body's circadian rhythm to the external cycle of light and darkness.

- The basal forebrain, near the front and bottom of the
brain, also promotes sleep and wakefulness, while
part of the midbrain acts as an arousal system. Release
of the chemical adenosine supports your 'sleep
drive'. Caffeine blocks the actions of adenosine.
- The amygdala, an almond-shaped structure involved
in processing emotions, becomes increasingly active
during REM sleep.

The stages of sleep

There are two basic types of sleep: rapid eye movement
(REM) sleep and non-REM sleep (which has three different
stages). During a typical night, a person cycles through
all stages of non-REM and REM sleep several times,
with increasingly longer, deeper REM periods occurring
towards morning.

- **Stage 1 non-REM sleep** is the switch from wakefulness to sleep. During this short period (lasting several
minutes) of relatively light sleep, your heartbeat, breathing and eye movements slow down and your muscles
relax with occasional twitches. Your brainwaves begin to
slow from their daytime wakefulness patterns.
- **Stage 2 non-REM sleep** is a period of light sleep. Your
heartbeat and breathing slow down and your muscles
relax even more. Your body temperature drops and
eye movements stop. Brainwave activity slows but is
marked by brief bursts of electrical activity. You spend

more of your repeated sleep cycles in stage 2 sleep than in other sleep stages.

- **Stage 3 non-REM sleep** is the period of deep sleep you need to feel refreshed in the morning. It occurs in longer periods during the first half of the night. Your heartbeat and breathing slow to their lowest levels and your muscles are relaxed. It may be difficult to wake you up. Your brainwaves become even slower.

REM sleep first occurs about 90 minutes after falling asleep. Your eyes move rapidly from side to side behind closed eyelids, your breathing becomes faster and more irregular, and your heart rate and blood pressure increase to close to waking levels. Most of your dreaming occurs during REM sleep (see page 256), although some can also occur in non-REM sleep. Your arm and leg muscles become temporarily paralysed, which prevents you from 'acting out' your dreams. As you age, you spend less time in REM sleep.

You need both types of sleep to digest the experiences of the day and transfer them to your 'memory bank'.

Briefly: sleep apnoea and narcolepsy

This book deals mainly with insomnia. But here are two further serious sleep-related conditions. They were treated at the clinic I attended.

Obstructive sleep apnoea (OSA) is a relatively common condition where the walls of the throat relax and narrow during normal breathing. This may lead to regularly interrupted sleep (and snoring) which can have a big impact on quality of life and increases the risk of developing certain conditions, including heart problems.

Narcolepsy is a chronic sleep disorder characterized by overwhelming daytime drowsiness and sudden 'attacks' of sleep. People with narcolepsy often find it difficult to stay awake for long periods of time, regardless of the circumstances. Narcolepsy can cause serious disruptions to your daily routine.

5th–6th November

0 HOURS, 0 MINUTES (SAY I)

335 MINUTES (SAYS THE SLEEP TEST)

WHAT?

I turn up for my assessment at around 6pm. A nurse shows me to a small room with a bed, a sink and an interesting-looking panel of electrical equipment on the wall. There is also a CCTV camera pointed at the bed, which initially freaks me out (it is to be turned on at 10pm, safely after I have changed into my night clothes). I make peace with the idea, I am here to be observed.

The nurse takes a swab to check for MRSA, then shows me into a sort of waiting room full of fellow patients, all in pyjamas. There's actually quite a jolly carnival atmosphere as I greet the narcoleptics, sleepwalkers and people with sleep apnoea. I seem to be the only person who is being treated for insomnia.

A chatty technician hooks me up to some extraordinary equipment, via electrodes attached to my hair with glue-like gel. It is akin to walking around with an octopus on one's head. The idea is that, once I am settled down for the night, this piece of technology will be attached to the panel in my room to measure my brainwaves. (These will reveal the amount of sleep I am having and its quality.) My octopus and I return to my room. I am advised to take my regular sleep medication.

Then, I cheat. I'm ashamed to admit this – and it was really stupid – but I did it. I have two nights' zopiclone laid out on the bedside table. When the nurse leaves the room, I take both of them.

I *know* this is somewhat counterproductive when I am about to be subject to a sleep study but, to me, this double dose represents a chance to maybe get some sleep (my pills are kept under lock and key at home). I justify it as a starving person might explain that they were so hungry, they ate two pies instead of one.

I am absolved on the grounds of necessity.

When the nurse comes back, she hasn't noticed. She tells me to go to the loo because once I am 'hooked up' I won't be able to visit the toilet until 8am without calling someone in from the night shift to extricate me. I panic. As many (mainly females?) may agree, there is nothing like a weeing restriction to make you want to go to the loo, like, all the time. I wee twice and then submit myself to the final bit of kit: a clip under my nose to measure my breathing.

Lights go out at 10pm and I prepare myself for the night ahead, trying not to notice the red blinking light of the CCTV camera pointing in my general direction. The gear on my head is heavy and I find the nose clip very uncomfortable. I need the loo all night long.

The extra tablet hasn't made the slightest bit of difference.

Several hours later, I watch the pale dawn break from behind the inadequate curtains. At around 8am, I am unhooked from the octopus. I have a quick shower to try to get the glue-like gel from out of my hair and go down to the 'dining room' (a conference room, really), to enjoy a breakfast of mini cereals and orange juice.

Eventually, the consultant comes in with a printout of my brainwaves. The polysomnogram maintains that I have, in fact, spent 335 minutes asleep (over 5 hours!), up to 4.37am, and much of this had been 'good quality'. THREE HUNDRED AND THIRTY-FIVE MINUTES?! To say I am surprised about this is something of an understatement.

My face must have said 'really?' as the consultant makes sympathetic noises about chronic insomnia being a difficult and intractable problem. I fess up about the extra pill but he shrugs it off and says that won't have really made any difference to the duration of my sleep.

The doctor continues by going through some basic (to me) chat on 'sleep hygiene' (e.g. no coffee after lunchtime, make sure your room is the right temperature, don't watch your iPad immediately before bed). As a reasonably intelligent person who has been suffering from severe sleeplessness for the best part of a decade, I had hoped for something more sophisticated.

I leave with a sense of frustration, a lack of solutions and blobs of gel in my hair, which take days to wash out.

14th December

0 HOURS, 0 MINUTES

A letter eventually arrives from the specialist saying that I have 'significant sleep state misperception' which 'often arises from a prior history of severe insomnia'. Perplexed, I feel I can't query the science. And I am so deranged with exhaustion, I almost don't care.

Maybe the mental health worker's approach is the only workable solution.

Accept you are never going to sleep again, Miranda, and move on.

PART THREE

Opening the Curtains

Year Eight

15th December

How could it possibly be that a bunch of machines can tell a person they have slept when that person knows for 'a fact' they have not?

Am I a phoney? A fraud? Suffering delusions, as the private psychiatrist insisted? Should I flush this manuscript down the loo, ask for some more olanzapine and a season ticket to the NHS nuthouse where I can start writing the missing front half of the Frank Sinatra biography?

I don't know. So I put on a Netflix film about Israeli spies.

Year Ten: A note from the future

Thankfully, I decided against the permanent throw-away-the-key option.

And, looking back, I have some questions for the sleep clinic.

The facts say I slept for 335 minutes. But who is to say what is 'fact' or 'science'? Objectively (from the outside), the polysomnogram told me I had slept for over five hours. Subjectively (in my experience), I have been awake all night.

Which verdict is the most meaningful: the subjective or the objective one?

Who is even to say what sleep 'means'?

We don't have the philosopher John Locke here, or even Professor Schrödinger and his cat. But it's time to ask some questions.

Sleep scientists . . .?

I revisit the consultant's letter. It doesn't shed much light on this conundrum. So I decide to call him at the clinic.

The doctor kindly agrees to speak to me. On discussing my diagnosis, he is engaged, not dismissive, as I feared he might be. 'The chart here is the pictorial report of an analysis of your brainwaves by technology,' he says. 'So you may have been getting more sleep than you thought.'

Just as my heart plummets, he adds: 'But maybe not. It's only the sleep we can "see". Sleep study is a young science and insomnia is a bit of a mystery. We are examining it to the best of our ability. In all honesty, problems like narcolepsy and sleep apnoea are easier to treat.'

Paradoxical insomnia, or sleep state misperception

According to the experts, sleep state misperception (SSM) is a term used for people who mistakenly perceive their sleep as wakefulness. There is also such a thing as 'positive SSM', where a person overestimates the amount of time they have been asleep.

While most sleepers with SSM will report not having slept in the previous night at all or having slept very little, clinical recordings generally show normal sleep patterns. Says the literature: 'Though the sleep patterns found in those with SSM have long been considered indistinguishable from those without, some preliminary research suggest there may be subtle differences between them.'

Back to Professor Guy Leschziner, the consultant neurologist who runs the Sleep Disorders Centre at Guy's Hospital.

Miranda: What's more important, Professor Guy? The objective 'results' or the subjectivity of how much a person thinks they have slept?

Professor Leschziner: The whole debate around SSM shows how we are poor witnesses to our own sleep. So which *is* more important? The bottom line is this: if you think you haven't slept but someone is telling you that you have, indeed, slept for six hours, that isn't going to make you feel any better.

M: So why did the machines tell me I had slept when I'm certain I didn't?

Professor L: There are two possible explanations:

1. We all have brief periods of waking up in the night, even for a few seconds. Your mental state at the time may have interpreted those few separate incidences as being awake for the entire time.
2. The second is, to me, the more plausible. At the clinic, you were attached to an EEG (an electroencephalogram) and four electrodes. These tell a doctor what is happening. But . . . only at a gross level, on the surface of the brain, not the whole of the organ. The brain does not exist in a unified state. Even while a person is awake, small areas of their brain are dipping in and out of sleep.

The sleep study therefore provides very limited information about your brain activity. It may well be that certain areas of your brain were awake and aware all night long.

As the science stands right now, we have no idea about the deeper structures of the brain. It's like trying to map the floor of the world's oceans using only a snorkel and a mask. You can only see one metre below the surface.

One person may have the same brainwave chart and say, 'I slept well.' Another might say, 'I didn't sleep at all.'

M: So, it could still be true that I didn't sleep for years on end?

Professor L: It's clear that you did sleep. If you didn't, you would be dead. It seems to me that you had local sleep in parts of your brain but also that parts of it were awake at the same time.

M: So if the machines can't define sleep, what is it exactly?

Professor L: Sleep is a result of a multitude of factors: the physiological, the neurological, the psychological and the environmental. The underlying biological process is very complicated.

I personally dislike the diagnosis of paradoxical insomnia. It implies the patient is bonkers. What is the point of telling someone 'you are clearly wrong' when they are complaining of terrible sleeplessness? It's not going to help anyone.

M: It's all still a bit of a mystery, isn't it?

17th December

SEVERAL MINUTES HERE, AN HOUR THERE

Something a bit odd, and not-altogether-unwelcome, is happening.

There are a couple of hours on the occasional night that I can't account for. For the past eight years, I could have told you exactly what was happening at any given point: there was continuity in the early-hours radio shows, for example.

But, increasingly, I've noticed the odd time jump. For example, I'll look at the clock, and it says 2.45am. The next time I glance, it might say 4.06. My usual point of despair is hearing the newspaper lady's car at 6.30 or so. Once or twice, I don't hear her at all.

I don't know why this is. And it should be amazing. But the problem is that I don't feel any more coherent or any less exhausted.

It seems pretty pointless to tick off these digits when I still feel like hell. But I must be sleeping. I must be.

Mustn't I?

18th December

2 HOURS, 3 MINUTES

I have got into the BBC quiz show, *Pointless*. I watch it religiously and am becoming a little obsessed. The celebrity version on Saturdays gives me even more of a *frisson*.

At 5.15pm, I come downstairs, pour myself a glass of red (I don't care about medication interactions – what's the worst thing that will happen, I'll get sleepy?) and watch Xander and Richard do their cosy, good-natured schtick.

Though my reactions are slow, I can even get some answers right – especially if they are on literature or history. I learn that Californium and Einsteinium make for good pointless periodic table elements, as does Djibouti, for questions about countries. I ace the word rounds.

Somewhere inside me is the faintest stirring of pleasure. Even if I don't want to admit it.

19th December

2 HOURS, 12 MINUTES

A trip to Dr F.

The appointment feels a bit same-old-same-old. But then I peek at the report he sends to the GP, of which I receive a copy.

'Miranda seems slightly more positive and her mood is definitely more lifted,' it says. 'There remain symptoms of depression including low mood, low energy, low motivation. There is equally report of poor sleep – she does not sleep more than two to three hours a night and does experience daytime tiredness. But her concentration is better. She watches quiz programmes on TV and is able to follow this through.

'However, Miranda does not feel confident linking up with her friends because of her weight gain. She eats well but perhaps more than she would have wanted and thinks this is due to the olanzapine. I also think her weight gain may be due to the olanzapine.

'I have brought to Miranda's attention that her level of activity is very low and definitely contributory. She took this on board.'

I agree with Dr F's verdict on my weight but don't entirely understand his optimism. Apart from those nanoseconds of delight when I work out the *Countdown* conundrum or know the *Pointless* answer, I don't feel better in the slightest.

Year Nine

5th January

2 HOURS, 47 MINUTES

Some family come over and Dad says there is a popular film we will enjoy. He puts on *The Greatest Showman*.

A few minutes in, I feel . . . something. It isn't positive. This film is the biggest pile of politically correct, mawkish, saccharine, forcedly feel-good vomit I have ever seen.

The 'something' I am experiencing is an opinion. It's one of the first opinions I have had in almost nine years.

Tarantino-film-liking, Chloé-shoe-wearing, ex-tabloid reporter Miranda would have hated this film. And so, now, does the Miranda who is ten years wearier, several stone heavier and seemingly coming back to life.

It's not a light-bulb, singing-and-dancing moment worthy of a musical tribute in *The Greatest Showman*. But it does feel rather good.

27th January

3 HOURS, 17 MINUTES

My God, I am fat.

I have a date with the surgery nurse for a flu jab and she makes me weigh myself. I squint one eye open to look at the number, shut it again immediately and almost fall off the scales again in shock.

There is an elephant in the room, and the elephant is me.

I have gained two stone in about five months.

28th January

3 HOURS, 30 MINUTES

My 'sleep hours' are creeping up. It's not an exponential thing – some nights I'll sleep three and a half hours; the next, two hours, forty-five minutes, and vice versa – but the trend is upwards, and it fills me with a joy that is almost impossible to express.

I'm starting to clock the world around me. And while it is mostly shiny and exciting, awakening to yourself as an obese person is not. I can't get out of the bath without going onto all fours first and can no longer put on my socks without performing some strange contortionist act.

This is a red line for me. It would be humiliating even if I hadn't been a naturally slim person for the preceding five decades. And – unlike sleep, which comes and goes on a whim and can disappear with a snap of the fingers for years – weight is something you can at least try to control.

My first life target in the peri-insomnia world is to lose some weight.

I read up about olanzapine. The withdrawal effects don't appear to be as brutal as benzodiazepines. So I make the unilateral decision to begin cutting down. If I feel worse, I'll reverse the process. I'm going to eat more healthily. Now I am less of a gibbering loon, I shall ditch the ready meals, chuck out the Scottish shortbread and cook with fresh and healthy ingredients.

I also vow to start doing some exercise. I put on my hideous Velcro-strapped trainers and leave the house. It's only when I'm halfway around the block that I realize *I am outside all by myself*. This is a major achievement.

But the fact that I have to stop, panting, to catch my breath three times in one circuit, notsomuch.

15th February

4 HOURS, 2 MINUTES

Four hours!

My father has a creaky old treadmill. I put the machine on its lowest setting and gingerly step onto it. When I'm satisfied that the treadmill and I are not likely to crash down onto the floor below, I walk a bit faster.

There's a TV in the room and I research comedy shows I need to catch up on. *Flight of the Conchords* and *The Inbetweeners* particularly tickle me (and each show is only 20 minutes long, so it's doable to exercise for one episode). As I march, I hear a weird sensation in my chest: I do believe that's called a laugh. With a few hours' sleep, my sense of humour seems to be waking up, and stretching, and yawning.

Forty minutes of exercise – I try to do two sessions a day – better diet, a quick taper of olanzapine with no obvious withdrawals. Almost immediately the pounds start to drop off.

27th February

4 HOURS, 12 MINUTES

My life is now governed by the Four-Hour Rule.

The Four-Hour Rule was a discovery from the early 2000s when my babies – only 20 months apart in age – used to play a nocturnal wake-up relay race every 45 minutes. It's the insomnia version of the the Five-Second Rule – the hygiene 'excuse' where it's OK to drop food or cutlery onto the floor and presume it uncontaminated if you can retrieve it in under five seconds.

After almost nine years of suffering, I have worked out that four hours is my threshold for functionality. So, as a general principle, if I sleep more than four hours, I'm good to go. Less, then I'm a bit of a hot mess.

It's also not set in stone. When I'm on the four-hour borderline, I sometimes trundle over the line of incoherence and back again.

My days go something like this:

I go to bed around 10.30pm and wake at any time between 2am and 4am. This is somewhat earlier than the rest of the UK. My wake-up is sudden – as if a light switch has been turned on. It's not accompanied by the lovely doziness of old: that craving to grope the snooze button and fall back to sleep. My brain just can't do that. So I need to find something to fill the time.

As my sleep improves, so does my social life. I have some old friends now living in New York, LA and Australia, so we start to write to one another. 3.30 in the morning in London is 10.30pm in Brooklyn, so this works quite well. I have also rediscovered social media, which was only in its infancy before everything fell apart.

I have started chatting to a nice American writer who I 'met' on social media during a political discussion.

From my bed, via my laptop, I have met some fascinating people: writers, professors, doctors, lawyers. They have recommended some fantastic literature and music and TV. It's also sort of comforting that whatever time you wake up, Twitter is still banging away.

At around 4.30am, I'll get up, go downstairs and have a leisurely cup of tea while the house is quiet. I'll listen to some music (quietly): Chopin is a current favourite.

I'm starting to feel ready to use my brain again – but how? Surely I can't be a journalist again, after all these years? It's an industry that moves on quickly: the footprints you left in the sand are rapidly washed away by the tide of the next talented arrivals. I start to ponder how I might retrain.

For the rest of the day I muddle along, frequently taking exercise in the mid-afternoons, which perks me up a bit. Five o'clock is 'wine o'clock' – not as 'bad' as it sounds, given it's usually just one glass and that 5pm in my world equates to 9pm in most other people's timelines. The problem is that by seven o'clock, I have a slight hangover.

During the short evenings I generally talk on the phone, WhatsApp my friends or text my children and cook dinner for my dad. Then maybe some TV.

By 10.30pm I am shattered. I have a bath, take my pills, read for a bit and fall back into an all-suffocating black slumber. No dreams ever. I'm not quite sure why that is.

Four hours or so later, rinse and repeat.

15th March

4 HOURS, 40 MINUTES

An email arrives from my brother. It's only within the past couple of weeks or so that I've felt *compos mentis* enough to look at a computer screen. A friend of his – Dr C – has written the first three chapters of a novel and wants a 'professional' opinion.

Oddly enough, I am able to look at this text with a critical eye. It's not half bad. I am not an editor of fiction, by any means. But from my past experience as an editor of journalism, I can make some suggestions of what works in basic prose and what doesn't. I am even able to compose an email with constructive criticism.

My traumatic conversation with my husband, all those years ago, was a *Sliding Doors* moment that triggered an almost-decade of misery. Watching – and hating – *The Greatest Showman* was also a *Sliding Doors* moment, in the other direction. With Dr C's chapters, the train starts to move.

I can still do it! Read! Comment! I have some use on this planet! I can't exaggerate what this does for my self-confidence.

The next morning, I pick up a paper and watch the news on TV. I sit at my father's computer and start deleting the

60,000 spam emails on my email account, before I give up the ghost and open a new one.

I am reconnecting to the world.

25th March

5 HOURS, 12 MINUTES

I sign up for two online courses. One is in commercial copywriting – an area in which I can see myself making a living. The other – just for fun, a gift from my father – is a Start Writing Fiction course at the University of East Anglia, which has a good reputation for creative writing.

Tonight, I decide to call a few friends, some of whom I haven't spoken to for several years.

K says: 'Which Miranda?' before sounding incredulous, then overjoyed.

W goes into a mercurial cycle of crying, laughing and shouting: 'Don't you *ever* do that to me again.'

L says what many of them were perhaps thinking but didn't dare say: 'I thought you might be dead.'

I still don't want to see anyone because I'm so conscious about my weight gain (I know, I *know*). But I feel that day creeping closer.

2nd April

5 HOURS, 4 MINUTES

I ponder my 'recovery'. I still don't know the 'why' yet. It's certainly nothing to do with the pills I've been taking. I've been on the same doses for years and am pretty much *off* the olanzapine altogether, now.

All I know is how it feels. Those eight and a half years were like being chained to the bottom of a pond. From down in the depths, I could perceive a distorted version of life going on above the water but I couldn't see or touch it. A few months ago, the chains holding me down started to strain. Finally, they snapped and I was free. I swam up and burst, gasping, through the surface of the water and into the open air.

I can breathe again.

Now, the sky is brighter, my new bamboo sheets feel luxurious, wine tastes better, music prompts powerful emotions. But I need to watch against taking in a surfeit of oxygen, or suffering the 'bends' from coming up too quickly, and crashing back down again. I don't quite trust my good fortune.

I also need to avoid sounding like one of those annoyingly evangelical people. You know, the ones who bang on about their 'rebirth' until you want to strangle them.

19th April

5 HOURS, 20 MINUTES

With a good diet and a modicum of exercise I have lost a fair chunk of weight but have reached a plateau. I wonder about hiring a personal trainer. I had one in the past, when I was a fit little sliver of a thing. Do trainers 'do' obese people?

A friend of my father's gives me a name. K is tough, sunny and isn't fazed by my lack of mobility. She's also reasonably priced. We decide to start on a programme of twice weekly visits – mainly walking to begin with.

We discover some fields five minutes' walk away. Though I have to stop several times for breath, I manage to walk for an hour. I tell K about my car-crash decade. She doesn't scream or run away, which I consider a good start.

12th May

4 HOURS, 23 MINUTES

It's my 51st birthday (I seem to have skipped the ones from 43 to 50). I'm still feeling like a puffy, newborn chick but I wonder about having my first night out in almost nine years. H and S say they would love to accompany me, so we book a table in a local pub.

I apologize to H and S about my weight on the phone in advance, asking them that if they are alarmed, please not to show it. When I open the front door, I brace myself for cartoon-like shock. But my friends are kind (or just good actors). There are tears as we hug: hugs that go on for a very long time. H tells me that yes, I look a bit 'inflated' (thanks, H) but I look healthy and happy. She even uses the word 'beautiful'. I tell her that's ridiculous. But I'd be lying if I didn't admit it made me feel better.

On arriving at the pub, I'm still a bit nervous. But from the first minute we sit down, all this dissipates. My friends are warm, funny and gossipy. I have my first cocktail for years. Actually, waiter, can we have another round, please?

Embarrassed about my weight, I initially refuse to have a photo taken. In the end, I relent, as long as it does not go on social media, where I am still using a profile pic from when I was an editor, nine years before.

15th May

5 HOURS

I am getting straight As in my copywriting course and encouraging comments for my creative writing. My confidence in my work is growing rather more quickly than my social and physical self-esteem.

My friend T (remember the one who, way back, got the job I wanted on the health magazine?) is working on a new publication and wonders if I want to write something straightforward about bugs related to kids going back to school.

I decide to give it a shot. If it's awful, I can always continue with the copywriting route. But you know what? I really enjoy speaking to the medical experts again and sound plausibly intelligent. I hand in a not-too-terrible piece of work.

20th May

5 HOURS, 14 MINUTES

For years now, people have been encouraging me to write about what's been happening in my life. (Er . . . nothing?) Until a couple of months ago, I couldn't pick up a pen or operate a laptop. My 'recovery' is also so new that I fear giving it voice might piss off the Gods of Sleep, who will renege on their benevolence.

Then I read about a TV personality complaining about his insomnia. Poor diddums only missed a few weeks' sleep but, boy, is he whining. In the Insomnia Olympics, I'd be on the gold medal podium while he'd still be warming up.

My tale is more powerful and I want to tell it.

I call up a big, national paper that I last worked for 20 years ago. As luck would have it, the editor who answers the phone remembers me. I offer to write my story and receive a commission to write 2,000 words about my Insomnia Crash, for the day after tomorrow . . .

22nd May

6 HOURS, 1 MINUTE

. . . and, oh! It gives me a thrill. My brain sparks, my fingers fly, I write the thing in less than three hours. Any worries I had that articulating my experiences might sent me back-sliding prove entirely unfounded. Yes, this is an emotional project, but it is cathartic.

My article is an oversimplified account of a complex and awful time – and a bit sanitized because I'm not yet ready to tell the whole disaster movie to the entire world.

But the gist of the story is there. It's pretty damn personal. I think it's quite good. Fortunately, my editor agrees. The piece comes out over a double page, with a misleading photo of a young and fresh magazine-editor Miranda – and even some shots from 20 years ago, when I worked on this particular newspaper.

(A feminist friend takes me to task over the photography situation: she says I should be proud of my body and how I look now. I roundly – sorry – disagree.)

The night before publication, I joke to the editor that I'm so excited, I won't sleep at all. She sounds genuinely worried.

But I open my eyes six hours and one minute after closing them. It's the most I have slept in almost nine years.

25th May

5 HOURS, 17 MINUTES (AND A VICTORY LAP)

The article has done well, attracting compassionate comments from around the world. Yes, there is always the odd nasty online 'troll' – a new subgenre of humanity I hadn't previously known existed – but these bitter strangers are easy to ignore. It takes more than that to upset me these days. Some of these comments are so outrageously insulting, they make me laugh out loud. One gentleman calls me an 'international waste of space'. But hundreds of people identify with elements of my story.

Suddenly, everywhere I look, people are complaining about their sleep. I can't move for TV documentaries, newspaper pull-outs, magazine covers promising '10 Ways to Sleep Better Tonight'. One article says that the 'sleep industry' is worth £100 billion.

As I come around from the Insomnia Crash, I discover that bad sleep is 'trendy': this decade's food intolerance. And with our sleep trackers, we want to be 'better' at it. (See the section on orthosomnia on page 161.) And while we are on the subject of all these devices, in the years to come, purchases of trackers and smartwatches are projected to go through the roof.

According to researchers, lost productivity caused by lack of sleep costs the UK economy up to £40 billion a year. I see another rumour the NHS is about to release guidelines for the first time – that people should sleep between seven and nine hours a night.

I decide to start a blog and H, a journalist friend, tells me how to do this. And so, talesofaninsomniac.com is born.

After a few days, I think there might be something in all this.

Much of the existing 'sleep literature' annoys me. Some articles almost have a hectoring tone, constantly reminding us of how 'bad' it is not to sleep for the magic number of eight hours a night.

I want to scream: *This isn't a choice, you morons! I would sleep for ten if I could!*

Maybe my fellow sleepless co-travellers need something more honest, from someone who has been there but who also understands how to talk to experts and doctors, to share advice. So I get in touch with J, an editor who has supported my work for years. She now works on the *Daily Telegraph*. To my surprise and delight, she would like me to repurpose my blog as an online weekly column for the newspaper.

5th June

5 HOURS, 12 MINUTES

What turns out to be my last appointment with Dr F. The difference in the atmosphere is extraordinary.

Dr F immediately picks up on my smile (for the past nine years I've been shooting daggers of hell when entering a psychiatrist's office), my open body language and my chatter. Apart from celebrating my recovery, there's not a lot to talk about. In fact, Dr F spends much of the session on the computer looking at the photos which accompanied my newspaper article, wondering where they were taken.

But I do want to talk about the drugs. I'd been a bit nervous about revealing I'd come off the olanzapine without consulting him but Dr F is entirely unfazed. For now, we will stick with the trazodone and the zopiclone. My sleep is vastly improved – why rock the boat when there are no serious side effects?

My only concern is the pregabalin (for more, see page 209), which is increasingly bothering me. About two and a half years after I started taking it, pregabalin was reclassified as a Class C controlled substance in the UK (Class C includes the strong opioid painkiller tramadol, as well as anabolic steroids). This was on the back of publicity about how the drug was being abused recreationally in prisons, had become a problem in various parts of Northern Ireland and had led to several deaths. Practically, this reclassification made it illegal for GPs to supply pregabalin and gabapentin through automatic repeat dispensing: doctors now have to hand-sign prescriptions.

I tell Dr F that I'd rather not stay on a drug with these associations, which I have also read has significant withdrawal effects. I'm on 250mg at this point, which I take in the late afternoons. Having learned a lesson from the benzos, we agree on a slow withdrawal programme of 25mg a month over a year.

In his letter to my GP, Dr F writes: 'I'm very pleased with Miranda's progress. Her mood is better and her sleep is improving. She is looking into writing and making some money. She is currently asymptomatic in terms of depressive symptoms or pervasive symptoms of anxiety.

'Today I advise that we transfer Miranda back into primary care.'

I've been discharged! I am no longer Officially Mad!

10th June

3 HOURS, 53 MINUTES

Nine o'clock and I'm at the pub with another old friend. As the evening progresses, I'm starting to feel increasingly weird. I start to sweat and a mild headache comes on. When I get up to go to the loo, I feel sick and dizzy.

I've only had one gin and tonic, so it can't be the alcohol. We've barely finished eating – surely it's far too early for food poisoning? Then it dawns on me. I forgot to take my pregabalin that day. I tell my friend, I'm sorry, but we have to leave, now.

Luckily the pub is only just down the road and I swallow my pills the second I get home. But I continue feeling dreadful for at least another hour, so I take another one. Just before bed, I start to feel better. But I don't sleep very well. My night is broken and I'm awake very early.

I set an alarm on my iPhone for 'pregab time' so I won't forget again.

So what is pregabalin?

Pregabalin (or Lyrica) is a member of the class of drugs called gabapentinoids. It was licensed first in 2004 for the treatment of epilepsy, then for neuropathic or 'nerve pain'. When it became apparent that one of the side effects was that patients felt calmer, pregabalin was licensed for the treatment of generalized anxiety disorder (GAD), one of my many diagnoses over all those years.

But around this time, 'red flags' had also started appearing in the medical literature that pregabalin – and its milder younger brother, gabapentin – could result in problems around addiction and dependency. Anecdotal evidence suggests there could be hundreds of thousands of people suffering on these drugs, especially when trying to come off them. What's really galling is that – as with benzodiazepines – most were prescribed by their doctors.

And it's a crisis that is growing. According to a recent report, prescriptions for pregabalin and gabapentin are rising in England. Between 2013 and 2018, prescriptions for pregabalin increased 1.8 times, while 6.7 million gabapentin prescriptions were written in 2017/2018.

Pregabalin was initially lauded as the modern, less problematic version of the benzos (see page 29) but right from the off some experts saw issues with it. The drug works on GABA – a brain chemical which promotes relaxation, reduced stress and alleviation of pain. The brain can become dependent on the chemical process produced by the drug. So patients want to stop their pills, then realize they can't.

Some doctors are quite forceful in their appraisals of pregabalin. For one of my newspaper articles, I interviewed Professor David Healy, a famous psychopharmacologist, and the author of 20 books on psychiatry. He told me: 'I'd rather be stuck on Valium. It's easier to get off. Pregabalin is Valium on steroids.'

Can you imagine how I felt when I heard that? Of course it wasn't as easy as just 'stopping'. As with Valium, I knew that ceasing cold turkey was dangerous as it could lead to fatal seizures. So I made that withdrawal plan with Dr F.

Wanting to see how it was for others in my situation, I visited the Lyrica Survivors (Pregabalin Support) Facebook group, which has 10,700 members internationally. Pregabalin is a biiiig problem.

And this comes back to the issues highlighted earlier in this book. Prescription drug addiction/dependency (delete as applicable) is a massive worry. As I write, news is continuing to emerge about the difficulties some people have coming off anti-depressants, as well as benzos and pregabalin. I've also started to wonder whether the on-off-on-off-again approach my doctors also had to anti-depressants affected me, too.

One thing's for sure, there is a need for dedicated services for those addicted to prescription drugs and a new crackdown on overprescribing.

18th June

5 HOURS, 45 MINUTES

I go to the supermarket with S. She pays for the groceries by simply tapping her debit card against a machine without having to enter her PIN. I am astonished.

'Don't you know about contactless?' she laughs. 'You have missed so much. You are like Sleeping Beauty, waking up after a hundred years.'

This is quite funny, so I pitch the idea to the *Daily Telegraph*. Here's an edited version of what appeared:

'I've just woken up from a seven-year news coma – what have I missed?'

Imagine if you have been in a coma for seven years. You wake up and the first voice you hear is Alexa.

Due to almost a decade of mental health issues, I missed a lot of news, and general life information. But now Sleeping Beauty – as my friends like to call me – is catching up. Every day there are new nuggets to discover, from the funny to the upsetting to the merely mundane. Below, randomly, in no order of importance or seriousness, is a pick 'n' mix of the highlights.

Social media is king. Before I left the planet, Facebook and Twitter were pretty new and I had accounts on both. As the editor of a parenting magazine, I was followed by PRs who represented nursery product brands. The chit-chat from clever journalists and celebrities was also mildly diverting. Then I switched off.

Newly reborn, I am enjoying the verbal exchanges of WhatsApp and Facebook Messenger and funny hashtags. But what is the deal with Instagram and Snapchat?

I went out for a birthday dinner the other week. On the next table, two twenty-something girls were staring glumly into their mojitos. Every 15 minutes or so, they would throw their arms around each other, break into false jollity and take a selfie.

Is anyone past their teenage years really interested in other people's meals/pets/holidays, etc.? Surely it's just bragging. Which segues into . . .

Words/phrases like 'humble bragging', 'woke' (how apt), 'virtue signalling' and 'Cis-gender'. People are 'cancelled' for saying the wrong thing. Cancelled? Like a flight or a hair appointment? Can you reschedule them?

What the hell are vaping shops and why are there so many of them on my local high street? What happened to Nicorettes? Why so many coffee shops? And does anyone use those electric plug sockets for cars? What happens when it rains?

Tinder and Grindr and allied 'dating' apps. Bit grubby.

Nobody talks to one another anymore. One friend says that every time her mobile rings, she knows it's me, because I am the only person who calls her (she is 49, not 15). How did this happen?

Everyone has a 'mental health' diagnosis. It's wonderful that there is less of a stigma allied to psychiatric conditions, that people are more open and accepting of each other. The change in the past ten years has been remarkable. According to a glossy magazine editor friend of mine: 'We start the day by comparing side effects from our anti-depressants.' And I think social media is a force for good in this aspect.

But there does seem to be a bit of a bandwagon. I remember when Catherine Zeta Jones was diagnosed bipolar and it was 'fashionable' for a while. Now everyone seems to have ADHD, or dyslexia, or cyclothymia. Even Princes William and Harry have weighed in.

While this is all laudable, severe, untrendy mental health conditions such as schizophrenia and manic depression (the pre-decimal term for bipolar) deserve to be taken seriously and allocated appropriate resources.

The utter dependence on WiFi. The modern life support system. We need these invisible airwaves for everything from communicating to buying clothes and food and ordering Ubers to travel around in. When we can't get the little stripey inverted cone on our devices, we become stressed, upset and violent. It's only going to get worse. Those without WiFi will be silenced, cold and will probably starve to death. The world will be ruled by BT engineers and those who know how to fix the broadband.

When I was last in the world, only hardcore football fans really had Sky. Now, 'normal' TV is largely rubbish. But once you tot up your BBC licence fee, Prime, Netflix and BT Sport (when did our phone company suddenly become a sports channel?) it's all getting quite pricey.

Why are £10 notes made of plastic?

21st June

5 HOURS, 10 MINUTES

I submit my final short story assignment to the fiction tutor. There is no grade but I can tell from her comments that she's pleased with my efforts.

1st July

4 HOURS, 55 MINUTES

Four to five hours' sleep is enough to function. I can speak, think, leave the house, enjoy things again. Compared with any time over the past nine years, it's a miracle.

But I am still tiiiiiiired.

I wonder whether there is anything that can boost me up to the next level, at least somewhere approaching that magic number of eight hours. Noodling around online, I come across something called cognitive behavioural therapy for insomnia (CBTi). Sigh. I had tried CBT (without the i) a few times during my Insomnia Crash. And it was hopeless.

Even so, it is unusual to see something with a dedicated 'i' in the title. I decide to find out more.

Cognitive behavioural therapy for insomnia (CBTi)

CBTi is defined as a structured programme that helps people identify and replace thoughts and behaviours that cause or worsen sleep problems. The idea is that you replace them with 'healthy' thoughts and behaviours that promote sound sleep.

Sleep guru Dr Sophie Bostock is an expert in CBTi. She says: 'CBTi is definitely more effective than drugs with none of the negative side effects. It aims to give you a set of "tools" with which to tackle your sleep problem. One set of tools is physical (behavioural) and the other is psychological (cognitive).

'People with insomnia need to reconfigure their routines, then change their view of sleep. There are several ways of doing this.

'**Sleep restriction:** This means spending less "quantity" time in bed for better quality sleep. So, only go to bed when you are tired and get out when you're not. Going to bed later increases your natural drive for sleep. In the short term, you can feel really tired but this often means a less broken night.

'**Stimulus control:** The idea is to strengthen the link between your bed and sleep in your mind. So use your bed only for sleeping, or sex, and nothing else. (If you've always slept with a TV on, and the thought of falling asleep without the TV makes you anxious, keep it on for now.)

'**Follow the "quarter hour rule":** If you are in bed for 15 minutes and still wide awake, rather than getting frustrated, you should get up, stop stewing and go and read a book. (TV is not recommended because it might stop you feeling sleepy. Mindless violence may not put you in the best mindset for a contented sleep and the "blue light" from a phone or a tablet can interfere with melatonin – the hormone in your brain that promotes sleep.)

'**Relaxation and mindfulness techniques:** We also teach clients various tricks and tools to help the brain to switch off its "fight or flight" response to stress. Since the mind and body are interconnected, relaxing the muscles can be a shortcut to easing the racing mind. For example, progressive muscle relaxation involves deliberately tensing and then releasing the major muscle groups in turn.'

These examples are great, I tell Sophie. But what if – like me, ten years ago – you are not sleeping *at all*?

Says Sophie: 'For people with very severe insomnia, I recommend forgetting about the cognitive part to begin with. Research shows that simply "BBT" or brief behavioural therapy can be effective.

'I always recommend starting with a sleep diary. If you are exhausted, you may find it frustrating, but it's hugely valuable. A journal puts you in the here and now and is a solid baseline. There may be complicated reasons behind your insomnia but a good routine is vital to build up "sleep pressure" – the compulsion to drop off. If your routine is haphazard there is no way you'll get a good night's sleep.

'So. Forget about bedtime for now. Set your alarm for 7am and get up, however you are feeling. Try to get outside as early as you can: morning light is really good for moderating your circadian rhythm. There is a lot of talk about sleep hygiene (see page 27). Clinical trials show that it doesn't make a lot of difference on its own but a much-cited paper does suggest it's best not to have caffeine within six hours before bed.

'Instead, follow a healthy lifestyle. Exercise, eat well, use your brain and relax when appropriate. People tend to roll their eyes when I say this but hearing this advice and nodding is rather different to putting it into practice.

'Go to bed when you feel sleepy. It doesn't matter if you wake up during the night. Your sleep goes in 90-minute cycles and people tend to wake up more as they get older.'

NOTE: *There are dedicated therapists who offer CBTi but they are few and far between and can be expensive. Digital solutions are now appearing. But many of the principles of CBTi are common sense. You don't need a therapist, or an app.*

You don't have to suffer from full-blown insomnia to benefit from CBTi. It can be useful even for the odd night when stress is making it hard for you to fall asleep.

7th July

5 HOURS, 12 MINUTES

I start to think about CBTi and how to apply it to my current sleep situation.

It makes a lot of sense, but I still question whether these practical issues could have helped me in the worst Insomnia

Crash years when I was incapable of following even the simplest instructions.

But now, with a few months of sanity under my belt, I think there are some principles I can apply to my current behaviour. Some of these I am doing naturally anyway – getting natural light, for example, and not having naps. But the idea of sleep restriction appeals.

And so I start going to bed at midnight, as opposed to my customary 10.30pm – and only when I am ready to sleep. I wish I could say I didn't look at my phone before bed, but, well. Hmm. Does switching off the ringer count?

I don't immediately start sleeping for longer but my waking hours have shifted. So instead of 10.30pm to 3.30am, I am doing midnight to five. It's still earlier than everyone else but is a bit more conventional. This knocks on – I get tired later in the day and can enjoy a more 'normal' evening, with energy to do more than just lie in a puddle in front of the TV.

I've also discovered lists. Initially, I used my lists as a 'brain dump' before bed, so I didn't keep ruminating on what I had to do the next day. But now, I love lists. No: I adore them. I write them all day long, on pieces of A4 paper I Blu-Tack above my desk. The lists have to be hand-written – somehow, doing them on the computer isn't the same. Then I colour-code them with marker pens: pink for work; green for social life, and so on.

Crossing things off my lists gives me enormous satisfaction, even if I never quite complete them.

11th July

5 HOURS, 29 MINUTES

I have lots of energy when I first wake up. I'm taking on more newspaper and magazine commissions and find that I get the most writing done between the hours of 5 and 10am. Sadly, my copywriting course has bitten the dust as I got back into my journalistic groove.

There is something magical about this time of day, enjoying the quiet hours before the world wakes up. When I was in the depths of my Insomnia Crash, I read an article by the ever-contrarian columnist Julie Burchill, who also suffered with sleeplessness.

She celebrated her insomnia – even going as far as calling it 'Extra Life'. At the time, I thought she was mad and that the statement might be a bit of a pose.

But now I am starting to understand what she means. OK, early waking after even just a few hours of refreshing sleep is not *quite* the same as insomnia. But it certainly provides more hours to get shit done.

Early bird or night owl? What is your 'chronotype'?

How long you sleep and when you wake is largely down to your genes. (Unless you work the night shift and you don't have a choice.) And scientists have been looking into it.

A recent paper attempted to explain the differences between 'night owls' who stay up late and get up late and 'larks' who go to sleep early and wake up early. People are said to have different 'chronotypes' – for example, those who get up at 5am are called the 'extreme morning chronotype'.

So which chronotype are you?

Dr Sophie Bostock has a suggestion for how to find out. Pick a run of days when you don't have any work or early social commitments. Go to bed only when you are tired, and wake up naturally, without using an alarm. 'We all have an inbuilt circadian rhythm which keeps our body operating on a 24-hour cycle of activity and recovery,' says Dr Bostock. '"Chronotype" is the term given to describe our natural time preferences for waking, activity and sleep. Most studies suggest there is a bell-shaped distribution, with fewer people at the extremes and the majority of people in the middle.'

Scientists believe our body clocks are programmed by genetic code but they are designed to adapt to our environment and change as we get older.

So, for example, children and the elderly tend to be early birds, whereas teenagers have a delayed clock, which means it is genuinely difficult for them to go to bed early or wake up early in the morning. It is estimated that, up to the age of 50, men tend to have 'later' chronotypes than women.

All well and good, but what if you have a 9 to 5 job and your chronotype sends you to bed at 3 and wants you to lie in until 10am?

'Our best guess is that a maximum of 50 per cent of our chronotype is down to genetics, so we definitely have scope to change it,' says Dr Bostock. 'While you might be predisposed to waking up at the same time as your parents, recent research suggests that you can adapt to a new routine by managing the things you *do* have control of – especially light and food.'

For example, a study published jointly by Surrey and Birmingham Universities explored what happened when 22 night owls, who typically woke up at 10.15am and went to sleep at 2.30am, adopted the behavioural patterns of earlier birds for 3 weeks.

They were asked to do various things, including going to bed two to three hours earlier than usual, recalibrating their alarm clocks to a similar time and sticking to the same sleep–wake schedule on work days and weekends. Subjects were told to have lunch at the same time each day and avoid eating dinner after 7pm.

After three weeks, participants had faster reaction times and a shift in peak performance from evening to afternoon. Perhaps most importantly, they had an improvement in their health, with lower overall levels of stress and depression.

15th July

5 HOURS, 46 MINUTES

As quickly as I spiralled down all those years ago, I am now looping back up. Things I *knew* I would never do again – well, I am doing them. Often effortlessly.

That 'getting back on a bike' analogy keeps coming to mind; except I'm still a bit fat for a bike and would probably wobble over and crash into in a heap.

These things include:

- Driving: I hadn't driven a car since moving back to my dad's. First it was a loss of confidence, then I thought I wouldn't be able to see well enough after my eye ops. Several tests reassured me that I had 20/20 vision with my specs on.
- Travelling on public transport: I thought I would be a quivering jelly the first time I stepped onto the London Underground. But when the train arrived, my brain kicked into Pavlovian gear. Elbows out, gimlet eye on the seat I wanted, taking no prisoners. The whole experience gave me enormous pleasure. The pleasure of the 'normal' that most people take for granted.* I was practically grinning.**
- Dropping under (cough, stone, cough, pounds) on the scales: Losing weight is really difficult, isn't it? Joyless and boring. But I am getting slimmer, if not at the pace that I'd prefer. I've learned that it helps to weigh myself at 5am, naked, without my glasses and with dry hair (it weighs more when it's wet).
- Dreaming: I have started to dream again. Not very often, it has to be said. But when I do dream, my night-time visions are vivid.

* Note from the future: This soon wears off.
** I'm not grinning any more, either. People were starting to move seats.

8th August

5 HOURS, 13 MINUTES

A reminder not to take my 'recovery' for granted and that I still need to take care.

Tonight, I have agreed to meet my friends K and J for dinner in a trendy part of the City of London. K is coming in from a different part of town, while J works in the area and will go straight to the restaurant. The travelling part no longer bothers me – I only have to sit on a train – but I am a bit nervous about finding the way to a new restaurant on my own. K offers to meet me at the Tube ticket barrier at Liverpool Street Station, so we can walk the last bit together.

For reasons K can't control, she is 25 minutes late. She is normally really reliable but because there is no reception on the Tube, she can't call to update me and I can't get through to her.

After a quarter of an hour hanging around by the barrier, I'm starting to get a bit antsy. This is peak commuter time, and workers are flowing up the escalators and swarming all around me. I call J – she has been waiting in the queue but is now being seated by the waitress. She says I should text K to tell her I'm leaving and come to join J at the restaurant. J tells me to use Google Maps (I have no idea what Google Maps is).

Stepping out onto the main concourse of Liverpool Street station is terrifying. I have not seen so many people in nine years and they are closing in on me from all angles, marching at great speed in that way of single-minded commuters the world over. I can't even cross the lanes of 'traffic' to get out of the way.

Remember Tippi Hedren in Hitchcock's *The Birds*? I have some empathy. (It doesn't help that I've broken my glasses, so my vision is distorted.)

I start to panic. This is not a sensation I've had since those office days at the start of my Insomnia Crash and it's actually more frightening. As I desperately seek the loo (in what you really would call a blind panic), I feel myself starting to cry.

There is a massive queue of blank-faced business people and tourists outside the toilet so I spin on my heels, looking for a different refuge. J calls: 'Where are you?' When she hears how distressed I am, she tells me to leave the station – but I can't find the way out. The layout of the concourse is so confusing, the blood has left my brain and I am incapable of rational thought.

In the end, J patiently 'talks me down' and helps me locate the escalator that leads to street level. I am hugely relieved. When she gently intones: 'Now, see the steps that are moving? Stand on the steps and get off at the end,' I can't help but laugh. By the time I emerge onto the city streets, I'm feeling a little more like myself again. But I'm still shaking a bit. So I jump into a taxi, even though it's only a ten-minute walk to the restaurant.

On arrival, I am angry with my friends for being so casual with me. I order some wine, finish it in one and slam the empty glass on the table. K arrives, bursting with apologies and tales of domestic delay – I tell her how annoyed I am. Both my friends are mortified. 'We thought you were doing so well,' they say. 'But clearly we forgot how new this is for you.'

I accept their apologies and we go on to have a lovely evening. But this incident reveals that even though my recovery seems amazingly fast, for a while, at least, it's two steps forward and half a step back.

10th August

4 HOURS, 30 MINUTES

I feel a bit guilty for shouting at my friends. My irritation was perhaps justified – but I know I am less patient and more moved to moods than I used to be. I know this is mainly because I am still very tired.

Why lack of sleep turns you into a toddler who missed a nap

Emotional niceties evaporate when a person is exhausted, with the body focused entirely on basic functions. Which apparently do not include whose turn it is to pick up the kids and where is my phone charger, please?

If you've had an insomniac night, the amygdala – the part of your brain that regulates emotions – starts to misbehave. In other words, sleeplessness turns you into a three-year-old, who overreacts and can ignore other people's feelings. And this can lead to fights which throw shade on your relationship.

I spoke to Susan Quilliam, a relationship expert and coach I've been consulting for my articles for over 25 years. 'When meeting new clients, one of the first things I do is ask whether any practical challenges in their lives might be contributing to their relationship problem,' she says. 'Often, when such practicalities are cleared up, the more emotional problems resolve themselves. So, if someone has sleep issues, I suggest they sort them out.'

Quilliam accepts that with insomnia, this is often easier said than done. However, 'it's hard to overestimate the devastation caused by a lack of sleep,' she says. 'Your anger levels go up, as does your anxiety, and your ability to solve problems plummets. You go into "meerkat mode", on full alert for danger. And if your partner makes you feel threatened, things go downhill swiftly, leading to a defensive response.' Cue the carnage of the last straw and angry words in the heat of the moment, often not meant.

So what should you do? First, a very practical piece of advice. 'If you find yourself in a hostile confrontation, leave the room,' says Quilliam. 'Not for three minutes, or five, but at least twenty, maybe even for half an hour. That's how long it takes for your adrenaline levels to subside. Then you'll be able to have a more reasonable conversation.'

Quilliam's advice is around 'emotional regulation'. 'It can help to take yourself out of the "feeling mode" and into "acting",' she says. 'If you feel the situation with your partner deteriorating, say: "everything will be ok, but I need to go and do something else for a while." Then find something calming to do.' This could be as simple as having a cup of tea, going for a walk or listening to a meditation app. 'I tell clients to develop their own strategy and then to write it down so they can read it in the heat of the moment, when they can't think straight,' she says.

Assuming you will eventually calm down, it's then important to make time for your partner. In the immediate term, this means doing your best to stick to any social plans you have made, however tired you may be. Moping about at home feeling shattered means that arguments are probably far more likely to start; taking you 'out of yourself' can also distract from your exhaustion.

15th August

5 HOURS, 49 MINUTES – AND FREE STUFF!

Work is going well and 'The Insomnia Diaries' column is proving to be great fun. I persuade my editor to let me do a 'tried and tested' of products that are supposed to help you sleep.

Not only will I get a whole load of free shit, there might be something helpful in there, both for myself and for the readers. Here are a few things I tried/discovered:

Sleep robotics

Somnox the sleep robot looks like a big, grey, cuddly kidney bean. The idea is that you take this gadget to bed and he will 'soothe mind and body to help you fall asleep faster, sleep longer and start your day feeling fully recovered and energized'.

Somnox does not disappoint. He arrives with a birth certificate and I decide to call him Beany. The fact there is an instruction manual makes my heart sink but actually, it's easy to follow. And sure enough, Beany starts breathing.

There is something endearing about Beany, who sits next to me all day while I am working. I pat him every so often, and occasionally give him a kiss.

At my 11.30ish bedtime, I feel a bit silly taking a piece of quilted machinery to bed. I have disabled the 'ambient sounds' option because I'm not really a fan of wailing whales. Beany is reassuringly stolid, and we are breathing in sync. (You set up the breathing rate through the app on your phone before you go to bed.)

I don't actually sleep for more hours but I wake up feeling happy, and pleased to see Beany first thing. This feels like the surreal plot of a European art house film.

The downside is that Beany costs five hundred quid.

Weighted blankets

So, weighted blankets have been a 'thing' in the States for a while now. They are marketed as an aid to anything from insomnia to anxiety and ADHD, and even for children with autism or Asperger's. The blurb on my blanket says it's 'designed to be warm and to provide pressure to a person, mimicking the feeling of being held or hugged'. The scientific jargon is that weighted blankets work through imitating 'deep touch pressure' (DTP).

I haul mine out of the box – all 15lb of it. This has been a stressful day with a piece on a tight deadline for a newspaper. I shuffle onto the floor and (with a small struggle) pull the blanket up to my neck. The weight of the blanket immediately makes me relax.

The best way to describe it is to recall the feeling I had as a small child, tucked tightly into bed – so tightly I could hardly move – after a bath and a bedtime story, secure and loved; calm and happy. I'm not really a worrier these days, but I definitely feel less 'wound up' under my blankie.

Later in the year, I decide to try it for sleep – after all, insomnia is my thing. I manhandle it onto the bed. That swaddled-baby feeling is better than ever – and because it is late autumn, I immediately feel warmer, and can shed one of the tops I was wearing.

The first night is a bit strange and heavy, but from the next night onwards, I notice that I am sleeping for longer, unbroken periods (I usually wake up at least once during the night, and again around dawn). I wouldn't say my sleep period increases, but it feels deeper – and I reap the benefits the next day.

NOTE: *In summer, I feel a bit hot under my duvet and my blanket, and the blanket isn't quite big enough to use on its own (nor the bamboo cotton texture I like next to my skin). So I don't use it for sleeping then, but even in July and August I love being under my blanket at the end of the day, when unwinding in front of the telly.*

Recommend!

The sleep–wake light

A large electronics company sends me a sleek, donut-shaped piece of equipment that wouldn't look out of place in a house designed by Kelly Hoppen. Minimalist chic aside, this light is designed to 'gently prepare your body for waking up during the last 5 to 60 minutes or last period of sleep', and will help you be in a better 'overall mood' in the morning, and to enjoy more energy.

I set the clock for 5am, around the time I usually wake up naturally. My bedtime is 12.30am, a bit later than usual, so I really am fast asleep when the light eases into action. I probably should have moved my wake-up call back to 6am. But actually, it's rather nice being woken up by a gently 'dawning' light and the sound of jungle birds. I like this light and will certainly continue to use it.

Meanwhile, my bedroom is getting a bit crowded with all this kit. Is it time to kick Beany out of bed?

Cannabidiol (CBD)

You can't move in a health-food store or chemist these days for shelves laden with CBD products.

According to online literature, CBD is a component of the cannabis plant which interacts with your endocannabinoid system, which 'helps your body maintain a state of balance and stability, known as homeostasis'. The 'dope' component that makes you 'high' has been taken out.

Grand health benefits are claimed for CBD, including the relief of chronic pain and inflammation. Some research and anecdotal evidence also suggest that CBD can help you get a good night's sleep. For example, one small American study showed that almost 80 per cent of subjects who took 25mg daily of CBD reported lower anxiety in the first month. Two thirds said that they slept better.

Some commentators suggest that CBD is particularly helpful when the insomnia is caused by external factors, including pain or inflammation. To me, it all sounded a bit 'woo-adjacent' but in the interests of research I did try out various CBD products, from oil you take under your tongue and balms for the skin to chewy pastilles.

I have to be completely honest, here. Some of the products are luxurious – and the pastilles tasted nice – but CBD hasn't made a blind bit of difference to my sleep. It's also quite expensive. But others' mileage may vary.

A quick note on bedding

Mattresses and pillows

There is an alarming array of fancy mattresses known by their first names, like the protagonists of a Jilly Cooper novel.

Marketing literature suggests changing your mattress every eight years but there doesn't seem to be any health reason for that, beyond the bank balances of the mattress companies.

There is helpful advice out there. James O'Loan, superintendent pharmacist for Chemist4U, recommends keeping your mattress clean. When I interviewed him for an article I was writing in 2019, he said: 'Most people forget about washing their mattress because they concentrate on their sheets. However, you should be thoroughly cleaning (baking soda is a good cleaner) and vacuuming your mattress. Plus, it's a good idea to flip it over every month or so.'

Those who suffer dust mite allergies face a different set of problems. 'Eliminating house dust mites is very difficult,' says Professor Adam Fox, a consultant paediatric allergist at the Evelina London Children's Hospital. 'An allergy to dust mite faeces – bunged up nose, itchy skin – can seriously interfere with your sleep. It's like having flu all year round. The best thing to do is limit exposure to this allergen.

'I recommend that my patients buy occlusive covers that go all the way around the mattress.' (These keep out dust mites and can be purchased via the Allergy UK website, see page 284.) 'There is minimal research data on the effectiveness of hoovering your mattress,' says Professor Fox. 'But it certainly won't do any harm.'

Professor Fox also recommends DermaSilk pyjamas (see page 283). These are part of a range of clothing products to soothe those with eczema. A note, too, for those who still sleep with a cuddly toy: teddies are notorious harbourers of dust mite poo. This is not ideal from an allergy perspective, says Professor Fox. 'But if there's no way around it, put your teddy bear in a hot wash once a month. Failing that, an overnight stay in the freezer does just as well.'

Sheets

A recent survey revealed that a quarter of British people only change their sheets once a month. Eew. 'Results show that using the same bed sheets for four weeks leaves you sleeping in worse types and more bacteria than you would find in a chimpanzee nest,' reported the literature. Gag.

In response to this, James O'Loan had the following to say: 'It comes as no surprise that beds become breeding grounds for bacteria as the weeks progress. After all, from the outside, bed sheets look pretty clean as they don't come into contact with "hard mess" all that often.'

O'Loan suggests that not bathing or showering before retiring can turn your bed into 'a harbouring ground for bacteria. Allowing bacteria to harvest in your bed sheets can lead to complications including hay fever and even pneumonia.' Given most adults spend seven to eight hours in bed, and children up to twelve, it's really important to address these health issues.

So how often should you wash your sheets? 'I would suggest once a week (28 per cent of people in the survey did this), bi-weekly at least,' says O'Loan. 'Set your washing machine to a minimum of 60 degrees and use a bleach-based detergent. You should be washing your top pillowcases more frequently than this, because they have direct contact with your face, mouth and other sensitive areas.'

O'Loan also recommends using an antibacterial fabric disinfectant ('They are pretty cheap nowadays – less than £5,' he says). 'Use a disinfectant on your sheets every couple of days while you're between washes. This'll keep the bedsheets smelling fresh but will also keep the bacteria from breeding.' Just make sure you are airing out your sheets and not leaving them damp because humid conditions are also a breeding ground for germs.

17th August

1 HOUR, 24 MINUTES

Since my 'recovery', I have hardly dreamed at all. Nor have I had an A-grade bout of sleeplessness. But last night, I was fortunate to encounter both. Here is a diary of my first – for a while – *nuit blanche*, as the French like to call it.

1.34am: I wake up with a start. I have just had a horrible nightmare in which a man is attacking me with a machete. I am in a state of terror and despair until a kind doctor from Leeds (no, I have no idea why, either) promises that he can save my arm.

I'm so shaken by how real this dream feels that I'm not sure that I a) can go back to sleep or b) want to, in case it carries on. So I decide to go downstairs. I put on a Mozart piano concerto and make a cup of green tea.

2am: I call a friend in Los Angeles and tell her all about it. She (sitting in the late afternoon sunlight) puts my night-time traumas into perspective and suggests I try to get some more sleep.

3.15am: I go back to bed. But after 15 minutes or so I still don't feel sleepy, so I get up again. I know it's game over for this particular night.

I go online. Lots of chatter and some 'direct messages' from overseas friends, actual and virtual. It's comforting to know there are always people awake somewhere in the world. As night falls on America's east coast, Australians are getting ready to have lunch.

5am: Dawn starts to break. I make a coffee, some toast and eat a couple of fat Medjool dates. I go into the back garden. Standing there in a sweatshirt, cradling my coffee in both hands, I'm reminded of an old cinema advert where a girl does something similar, to the accompaniment of the song 'I Can See Clearly Now'.

I mention this on Twitter and within seconds someone has posted a link to a Nescafé advert called 'Sunrise', from 1988.

I send a tweet canvassing people for their favourite morning songs, then ask Alexa to play them. They include:

- 'Here Comes the Sun' and 'Good Day, Sunshine' by the Beatles
- 'Lovely Day' by Bill Withers
- 'Good Morning, Good Morning' from the musical *Singing in the Rain*
- 'Morning Has Broken' (Cat Stevens' version)

6.30am: I have a big, hot bath with L'Occitane Rich Foaming Bath.

7am: When choosing my outfit for the day, I decide to wear a white top because a fashion journalist once told me white is flattering if you look tired. Even though no one's around, I put on a bit of make-up and a soft, luxurious scarf I bought yesterday, because it makes me feel good. I'm bone-tired.

7.10am: Maybe some exercise will wake me up a bit. I decide to pop out and post my nephew's birthday card. It's good to have some fresh air and to see the morning. The post box isn't far away but I power-walk around the other three quarters of the block. It's really windy for August but kind of exhilarating. Good to use my muscles.

I almost step on the smallest snail I have ever seen.

8–11.45am: I wrap up some work loose ends (my brain is fried, so there's no point starting anything which requires logical thought) and do a bit of noodling around Facebook and Twitter. I know I should cut back on both of these. I talk (online, of course) to a few of my journalist friends about our adult social media addiction. We decide it's a real issue.

12pm: I go for a swim. Oh, it feels so good to lose myself in the water and stretch my muscles. As I knew would be the case, I feel far less mentally exhausted afterwards.

1.30pm: I catch the second half of Manchester City v West Ham, MacBook on my lap. I always find football relaxing. Nice, unthreatening men wittering on in clichés for an hour and a half or so. I suspect that not many people share this view, especially West Ham players and fans (they lose 5–0).

4pm: I hit a serious slump now – too tired to think straight at all. There's no point me having a nap – the only time in my life I ever slept during the day was when my babies did (and sleep deprivation caused by external factors is very different from insomnia or bad dreams caused by one's own brain). I start to worry that writing about insomnia and thinking about insomnia this much is, in fact, causing insomnia. What if I've had a good run and will go back to a long period of not sleeping at all? I feel stressed and unhappy.

5.30pm: It's early but I'm hungry and decide to cook dinner for my father and myself. Normally, I'd have a glass of wine or a gin and tonic at this point but I feel so rubbish that I don't think it would be a good idea.

The seared salmon, tomatoes in olive oil and sweet potatoes go down well and I rally temporarily.

6–8.22pm: Little bits of things: the Sunday papers, a phone call, some Twitter, another bath. I'm exhausted but I feel supported and strong, which is very different to how I felt when I became 'ill' with severe insomnia all those years ago.

8.22pm: Yes, it's super early but I can't keep my eyes open for another second. As I get into bed, I worry about how quickly I will fall asleep, if at all, and whether the marauding machete man will come back to get me. But . . .

. . . suddenly, it's 2.28am: I have slept deeply for six hours. Which is pretty much as good as it gets for me these days and I do fine on that. There is no point me trying to doze any longer because once I am awake these days, I am awake.

For today at least, I am back in the game.

23rd August

4 HOURS, 15 MINUTES

I know I am becoming more confident because I change my social media avatar and allow a more recent, tubby photo of myself to be published in an online article.

My feminist friend is pleased.

25th August

3 HOURS, 24 MINUTES

This week, there has been a heatwave like no other. Going outside is like walking into a wall of warm, wet towels.

The nights – for everyone – are pretty torrid. We insomniacs enjoy a little Schadenfreude because 'normal' sleepers are having a taste of what it's like for us, all the time. And, boy, do those tough bedroom warriors bitch and moan.

Here are some thoughts on surviving the sultry season:

DON'T put your pyjamas in the freezer or go to bed with wet socks. Apparently, both of these are 'things'. When you defrost, they will only make you soggy.

DON'T try to sleep. Imagine yourself instead on vacation with an American movie star. 'Whisk yourself away to a time and place when you can imagine enjoying lying in the heat – it could be real, it could be imaginary – a favourite beach, pool or sunlounger. Who is there? What can you hear? What can you feel?' asks my sleep guru, Dr Sophie

Bostock. 'You can use imagery to distract yourself from the current discomfort. Even if you don't get straight to sleep, at least (in my case) you can enjoy sunbathing with Bradley Cooper.'

DON'T take naps as they will disturb your circadian (day/night) rhythm. But siestas work for the southern Europeans.

DO apply cool, wet cloths or ice packs wrapped in cloth to your wrists, armpits or groin for short periods as these are areas where blood flows closest to the surface of your skin.

DO see your doctor if you are on diuretics (fluid tablets) as you'll need to check how much to drink in hot weather.

DO place a tray of ice cubes in front of a fan in your bedroom. (A note on fans: make sure yours isn't squeaky like mine is, so I can only use it during the day. It also blew away the receipts I had carefully arranged on my bed, for accounting purposes.)

DO kick your pets and your partner out of bed because animals and people are hot and sweaty and two of them doubly as hot and sweaty as one sleeping alone.

DO keep the bathroom light on all night, because you will need the loo. According to some experts, we should drink three litres of water a day. (But not more than one litre an hour, according to the US website Medical News Today, because of hyponatremia, a rare but nasty condition where you dilute the sodium in your bloodstream and become very unwell.)

DO get air conditioning. 'Totally worth it,' says my (UK-born) friend T, who lives in Los Angeles. 'The Brits do seem to resist the movement of air inside. I could not talk my father into getting a fan and he was always moaning about the heat. I finally bought him one and had it sent over. He loved it, of course, viewing it like some kind of mysterious modern miracle. When you have a/c it doesn't matter how hot it gets. It was 100 degrees here today . . . But in my apartment, almost chilly. And while we're on it, what's with the shitty washer dryers? And showers?'

Sleeping in winter

While we are on the subject of sleeping during a heatwave, what about those nights during the coldest months of the year? In winter, we crank up our thermostats, wear chunky jumpers and sit in front of roaring fires. But what happens when we crawl under the duvet at night?

'There tends to be more information on summer sleeping, because of the assumption it's easier to fall and stay asleep in a heated house in cold weather,' says Dr Sophie Bostock. 'But this isn't necessarily true.'

To understand sleeping in both extremes, we need to appreciate our circadian rhythm, and how our internal temperature changes throughout the day. 'We can see ups and downs every 24 hours in our core body temperature, heart rate, blood pressure, hormone production, reaction times and mood,' says Dr Bostock. 'We're biologically adapted to sleep undisturbed when our body temperature is at its lowest. This naturally happens in the early hours of the morning, before dawn.' The trick, then, is to find an optimum temperature in order to fall asleep.

This starts with your bedroom. 'The best temperature – regardless of the time of year – is between 18 and 21°C,' says Dr Bostock. 'For this reason, it might not be a good idea to have the central heating on all night. Most people have experienced hot and uncomfortable nights in a hotel with the heating blasting out. I prefer to keep the radiator in my bedroom switched off all day, as well as all evening: even in the winter.

'The core of our body moves towards sleep by sending blood to our extremities in a process called vasodilation,' says Dr Bostock. 'If we are too cold, this process shuts down. This is why a warm bath or shower before bed is a good idea. Cold showers or ice-baths will stress the body too much; a sauna will overheat your core.' Bostock points to a 2019 digest of 13 studies which claimed that warming the body for at least 10 minutes, an hour or two before bed can shorten sleep latency (the time it takes to fall asleep) by 10 minutes.

A hot water bottle by the feet or bedsocks can also be useful, says Bostock, but it's best not to risk overheating in bed – for example, by leaving an electric blanket on all night. 'If you get too hot, it will interfere with deep sleep and may wake you up. You're most likely to wake up in the second part of the night, during REM sleep, when you're less good at regulating your temperature,' she says.

The right temperature is vital, but it's just as important to regulate your intake of light during the darker months.

'Exposure to daylight can help you maintain restful sleep and a more positive mood throughout winter,' says American sleep expert, Dr Michael Breus. 'Light exposure first thing will inhibit melatonin production, and stimulates cortisol, the hormone that activates behaviour. This will give you more energy during the day and make it easier to fall asleep at night, with more refreshing, restorative rest.'

Says Dr Bostock: 'Many people have a delayed internal rhythm during the winter months. You need to coax your body clock back into gear. If you find it hard to get going, an early morning walk will wake you up, via melatonin and movement.'

15th September

3 HOURS, BECAUSE OF THE WEIRD JET LAG THING

Since my Liverpool Street panic attack, I've become much more proficient at travelling and crowds. I've been to Edinburgh by myself and into central London more times than I can shake a stick at, with no incident. In fact, I rather enjoy travelling alone.

One might argue that a trip to New York is a bit of a stretch for my first foreign trip since getting better but it's my favourite place in the world and I want to see it again. 'A life lived in fear is a life half lived' (as Scott Hastings said in Baz Luhrmann's film, *Strictly Ballroom* – and Baz knows all).

Anyway, I've missed enough years of fun, thank you very much, and I have several good friends in the Big Apple.

(I also want to meet the nice American writer. We have become rather close.)

I've decided not to write too much about my new romance in this book. But from the sleep point of view, I'm alright. Turns out, I'm rather used to wandering about in a semi-zombie state, so a minus-five-hour time difference is child's play.

Before leaving for the States, I take the opportunity to ask a long-haul expert for his tips and tricks on surviving the several-time-zone jump.

What you can learn about sleep from a long-haul pilot

To reach your exotic holiday location, you need to suffer the grime and ennui of a long-haul flight. Not only the boredom and bad food, but also (for most, except the lucky or the medicated) sleeplessness and a confusing romp through several time zones.

So, how does your captain stay responsive and alert? And can we apply this wisdom to our daily routine, whether we are flying or not? I spoke to a senior British Airways pilot. And, as ever, I asked my sleep guru Dr Sophie Bostock for tips on adapting to long-haul trips in our short-haul lives.

This advice might also be helpful for shift workers. In fact, it can be applied to many situations when you are moved out of your sleep 'comfort zone'.

Captain Charles Everett has been a BA pilot for 32 years. He currently flies the state-of-the-art A350.

Don't worry if you can't sleep

Captain Charles says: 'I plan four hours' rest before my wake-up call. If I can sleep, that's wonderful, but over the years I have taught myself not to feel anxious if I can't drop off.'

Dr Bostock says: 'This advice goes for everyone. The biggest enemy to sleep is trying too hard to sleep. If you accept that you might only be able to relax, it will still reduce your stress levels and improve your mood.'

Eat when you're hungry, sleep when you're tired

Captain Charles says: 'It's easy to overthink the effects of a long-haul lifestyle with complex routines. I like to be adaptable. But I do tend to eat light meals around the time I'm flying: salad with white meat, avocado or egg on toast. I drink lots of water throughout the day and when I'm in the air.'

Dr Bostock says: 'This is great advice. Listen to your body. Don't try to force sleep when you're not tired – it may be counterproductive. On the subject of diet, healthy eating is important at any time but especially when your body is under the stress of sleep deprivation. Try to avoid eating in the middle of the night when your body clock is less able to metabolize food. It's vital to stay hydrated.'

Take exercise you enjoy

Captain Charles says: 'Some of my younger colleagues have adventurous pursuits like kitesurfing; others do yoga or Pilates. I enjoy hiking, especially in California. It's good exercise but also social: there's always someone who wants to come along.'

Dr Bostock says: 'The relationship between sleep and exercise is reciprocal. Regular exercise increases your natural drive to sleep and relieves stress, while good-quality sleep gives you the energy to get active. Physical activity also signals to our body clocks that it's time to stay awake.'

Don't drink alcohol before an important day

Captain Charles says: 'A pilot is not allowed to have any alcohol in his or her bloodstream: it's against the rules. I never drink the night before a flight, not just because of random testing, which could happen at any time, but also because I don't sleep as well under the influence of alcohol.'

Dr Bostock says: 'It's tempting to have a drink if you're anxious about something the following morning. But if you have two or more drinks, the quality of your sleep will be worse and you'll wake up more tired and groggy than if you'd stuck to mineral water.'

Clear your mental inbox

Captain Charles says: 'A friend gave me some advice: "Never open an email unless you are going to deal with it or delete it." I don't always stick to this but do find that completing tasks – even trivial ones – can enhance meaningful sleep. To illustrate: I now have two days off after a trip to Dubai. I need to write a report and could put it off, but I want to get it done so I have a clear mind tonight.'

Dr Bostock says: 'Some people find it useful to write down their "must do tomorrow" list as they wind down for bed so that they don't keep ruminating on these thoughts whizzing round their head.'

(I say: You see, lists!)

Accept your limitations at 3am

Captain Charles says: 'For a flight, say, to the USA's west coast, there's normally a captain and two co-pilots on board, sometimes three. Pilots work in shifts of about six hours with three hours' rest, and we give each other a lot of support. Experience tells me that the period of "low circadian rhythm", at 3 or 4am, is difficult. I used to think the answer was coffee. Now, I just understand and accept what I am feeling, and ask a colleague for help if I need it. And offer it back.'

Dr Bostock says: 'We find it hardest to stay awake during the circadian low, which is the time your body temperature is naturally at its coolest and when you've built up a lot of sleep pressure from the preceding day. Short naps of 10–20 minutes can help pep you up if you need to be alert.'

Don't rely on caffeine

Captain Charles says: 'To wake up quickly, I'll splash water on my face and have a cup of tea – normally peppermint or lemon and ginger. Then I'll stand at the back of the cockpit until I'm alert enough to take charge.'

> **Dr Bostock says:** 'Highly caffeinated drinks mask the natural sleep drive, so you can't rely on how sleepy you feel as a guide to needing rest. More excellent advice from our BA captain.'

21st September

5 HOURS, 32 MINUTES

You may be pleased to hear that my visit to see the American writer went rather well.

My delight in this trip is not only about cementing my new romance, however. Pre-Insomnia-Crash me might have hesitated about flying to New York alone. Sleepless-for-years me would have told you you were out of your mind to even suggest the possibility.

But sleeping-again me loved every second.

Some examples of things I adored: buying a pre-dawn coffee at Blackfriars station and watching day break over the City while waiting for the Gatwick Express. Guessing the destinations of fellow passengers on the train. Feeling in my bag for my passport only five times an hour, instead of the customary twenty. The thrill of managing things *by myself* – going through security, finding the gate, setting up on-board WiFi. Not catastrophizing that the nice American writer wouldn't show up (he did) – but having a contingency plan, just in case.

And that's before we even mention Martinis in Midtown, dinner in Soho, walking the High Line, dashing around Brooklyn on an electric scooter before bagels and lox at Russ & Daughters. The confidence to enjoy an afternoon on my own in Williamsburg when said writer had business to attend to. Saying farewell after several days, but feeling happy and secure that we would see one another again. Even napping for a couple of hours across three seats on my return journey.

Because: this is freedom. This is life. These were the gifts that sleeping again (as well as being single again) had brought. This was my awakening.

Afterword

Year Ten
The Year of Corona

23rd March

6 HOURS, 10 MINUTES

I've been OK for over a year now. My life is pretty much back on track. I am just back from another NY trip when Prime Minister Boris Johnson makes his solemn, red-eyed speech announcing 'lockdown' because of coronavirus. I go cold all over. Yup, the COVID-19 situation is serious now.

But my immediate selfish thought is: *what about my sleep?*

Given that my near-decade of insomnia was triggered by a domestic crisis, what chance will I have with a world calamity?

I'm not feeling particularly anxious, funnily enough. But this is exactly the right time to revisit CBTi.

And in a time where you aren't even allowed to leave the house except for grocery shopping and one walk a day, routine is king. Here is mine:

Broadly speaking, I wake up to the *Today* programme, look at social media, have a bath, do some work, eat meals at regular times and make sure I do my allowed 'once a day' exercise: a 20-minute walk at least around some local fields. Fresh air is really important. Because we have less exposure to light in the autumn, winter and early spring, our circadian rhythm is affected and our body clock doesn't wake up properly. This means we are less likely to sleep well the following night.

Late afternoon, I start my evening routine. A wise therapist tells me to think back to when I was a child or had babies of my own. 'The routine was early tea, slow play, a bath, hot drink and bedtime story. Adults need their own version,' she says. Mine includes a glass of wine (um, OK, two), some TV and social media or phone chats.

I've started to enjoy cooking. It's like therapy, using a different part of my brain to the one that's on a computer all day. Later in the evening, I have a second warm bath with Epsom salts and a scented candle and NO *NEWS AT TEN*.

Upsetting news fires up anxiety, which is the opposite of what you need to fall asleep. The latest I will go is the *Six O'Clock News* but I'm starting to avoid that as well.

I'm doubling down on my 'sleep restriction' (see page 215), which, despite its name, is not about limiting the amount of time spent asleep but the time in bed doing other things which can interfere with sleep. So, I go to bed at around midnight and awake naturally at about 6am. I wake up at least once during the night and check my phone – bad! – but am fortunate enough to drop off back to sleep.

Things aren't perfect – on 'just' 6 hours I am often tired – but compared with 18 months ago, it's a revelation.

20th April

1 HOUR, 30 MINUTES – CORONAVIRUS DREAMIN'

At 1.30am last night, I sat bolt upright, sweating. I had woken from a dream where I was stuck in a tiny glass lift, so snug all around and so low above my head that I couldn't move and there was hardly room to breathe. A week earlier, a nightmare involved me trying repeatedly to phone my boyfriend to rescue me from some unspecified threat – but I kept dialling the wrong number (hundreds of times). Both were very unsettling.

I've always had dreams – both pleasant and not (see my machete dream on page 234) – throughout 'peace time'. But they do seem to be more vivid, and detailed, in the time of COVID.

I ask some friends if they've had similar experiences. Almost all agree. Some of them are hilariously surreal. Two examples: 'I had a dream last night that my friend had shrunk her husband to the size of a baby and was carrying him around.' And: 'We all went on holiday to a Soviet holiday camp and bumped into Kate Beckinsale who told me she was still married to my husband and was fuming she hadn't received the £28-million separation settlement.'

One acquaintance with left-wing sympathies dreamed she was having an affair with Boris Johnson – but only in order to bring down the government.

However, the majority report dreams based on domestic life that seem to show frustration, anxiety or fear: not being able to find the toothbrush, being in an out-of-control speeding car or having to sit an exam they hadn't revised for. 'I've been having very vivid dreams about being really late for work and getting into trouble with my boss,' says an editor I know. 'When I'm dreaming, it's almost as though I'm half asleep and I'm half awake. When I do wake up, it takes me a while to figure out whether it was a dream or something that actually happened.'

So what is going on here? It could all be that lockdown is just a fantasy and Boris will walk out of the shower in Bobby Ewing style and tell us it has all just been a dream. More likely, something interesting is going on in our brains.

Is there a science behind our dreams?

Professor Guy Leschziner is the clever neurologist from Guy's Hospital, London, who knows all about nightmares and other interesting nocturnal adventures. He says:

'Scientists believe that dreams happen in "active" REM sleep, as opposed to "normal" sleep. The brainwaves of a person in REM sleep look almost as if they are awake. The dreams we have in light sleep are bitty vignettes. But in REM sleep, they have more of a narrative structure.

'Sleep scientists hypothesize we've been getting more REM sleep since lockdown started and don't have to leave the house for work or the school run. We tend to do most of our REM sleep in the latter part of the night. Historically, most people are sleep-deprived: woken up before is natural by our alarm clocks. Now many of us don't have to get up early, we have REM rebound. We are all trying to make sense of the world right now. Dumped in this new environment, we are struggling to figure our place in it. The 24/7 news cycle doesn't help. You can't withdraw yourself from all news, but it's important to find balance.

'In "normal times", we are usually so focused on getting up and out of the house that we don't record our dreams. Now we have time to recall them, talk about them and write them down.

'And while some people report having pleasantly surreal dreams – or even none at all – many are having nightmares right now. But this may not be a bad thing. Dreams are a kind of overnight therapy. They are normal, not pathological. People with PTSD constantly wake up during the night. Therefore they don't adequately process their emotional experiences. And while certain people during corona-times may be traumatized – those on the front line seeing death on a daily basis, for example – most of us are haunted by a vaguer sense of invisible menace. This causes anxiety, rather than acute distress.

'So can we control our dreams? Not entirely, but we can reduce anxiety. Think about what relaxes you, whether it's meditation or mindfulness. Exercise helps, as does basic "sleep hygiene" – limiting caffeine, not going to bed hungry, keeping to a bedtime routine – and not watching the late evening news.'

But Professor Guy thinks our weird dreams might continue in a post-COVID world. 'Job insecurity and the continued health risk mean anxiety may persist in a lesser form. Prepare yourself for more interesting nights ahead.'

Common dreams: what do they mean?

'Dream interpretation does not have a strong basis in science,' says Guy Leschziner. 'Nor do dreams tell you anything specific about your life.'

But here, for fun, are some common theories gleaned from the Internet:

- Your teeth are falling out: represents anxiety about your appearance and how others perceive you.
- Being chased: suggests you are running away from something causing you fear and anxiety in your life.
- Unable to find a toilet: means you have trouble expressing your needs in certain situations.
- Being naked in public: symbolizes not being able to 'find yourself', or being wrongly accused.
- Not being prepared for an exam: a reflection of your lack of confidence and inability to advance to the next stage in your life. One in five people will apparently have this dream.

Present Day

As I come to the conclusion of this book, we are still in COVID peri-lockdown and face an uncertain future. Thanks to the Sleep Lords (and Ladies), I'm doing well in the zzzs department.

Some other nice things:

Work: This (touch wood) is going well. I'm regularly writing and editing for national newspapers, magazines and websites.

The drugs: I'm coming off the remaining medications – at my own pace. As it stands, I'm approaching the end of my pregabalin taper, but wild horses would not make me rush that. I'm still on the zopiclone, which purists may say is cheating/still being an addict but I don't give a shit!

No, it's one battle at a time with the medications. I will come off the zopiclone but in my own time. I'm also on the anti-depressant trazodone; I haven't decided what to do about that. The superstitious part of me doesn't want to rock the boat. And what is the rush, really? I'm thinking clearly and feel happy, healthy and creative. I guess there is always . . .

. . . **my weight:** But I'm also doing well, here. Somewhere between my olanzapine mammoth enormity and my fighting weight. My progress isn't dramatic but it's steady. I'm not dieting exactly, just eating healthily and exercising a fair bit. I'm still working out with K, the trainer – my favourite discipline is boxing with pads. It's fantastic for physical fitness and mentally satisfying to whack something, which helps get rid of frustrations. I feel fit and strong. I know I'm not going to be seven and a half stone again.

'**Style**': I'm taking care of my appearance again and have fully embraced the 'nail bar' culture (it's all about OPI's Malaga Wine varnish). Now I can fit into high street brands (and am earning a bit of money), I'm buying flattering clothes. Though I do love my satin M&S day pyjamas.

And, oh! Boots and shoes! How I love them again. The pink-trimmed Velcro trainers from Sports Direct stay in the cupboard as a testament to how far I have come. The Chloé Bay has just been upgraded to a Jérôme Dreyfuss Billy Bubble handbag.

'**Giving back**': After I interviewed Melanie Davis of the Change Grow Live REST group, she asked me to volunteer my time for a couple of hours a week. Which I now do, gladly.

That bloody personality disorder diagnosis: I had completely forgotten about that till I interviewed Dr Sami Timimi (see page 99). In the end, I called my GP, who said it was still on my records. She was slightly hesitant about taking it off but then I suggested she read newer diagnoses from different psychiatrists. Now, she assures me, it's gone without a trace. But this little story reveals how unwelcome labels can stick if you don't make a bit of a fuss.

Family and friends: Almost all the old ones are back, along with some lovely new ones to boot. I have also met some amazing professionals while writing this book and my related journalism.

I'm finally getting divorced. My relationship with my kids will probably never be the conventional mother/child one, given all we have been through. But it's delightful – and improving all the time. My daughter sadly won't be getting my wedding dress – thrown away in year five by the private mental health coach – but she does have my £400 Fenwick's leather jacket.

My relationship with the nice New Yorker continues to flourish.

On my 'self-development': If I was to fill in that empty gratitude form from the rehab centre, I would need two sides. Then I would ask for an extra sheet.

Since my Insomnia Crash, I've been told I have more empathy. I feel people's sadness and joy more keenly than I used to. I'm not sure if this is because I am older or because of what I've been through.

I'm not perfect, nor am I a saint – far from it. I'm still impatient and interrupt people because I'm in such a rush to get my thoughts out and I feel that I've lost enough time already. That can seem rude. I get annoyed by self-pity, unnecessary drama and hypocrisy – especially the latter.

People who can't laugh at themselves piss me off, as do 'energy vampires'.

'Fearless' isn't quite the word – who doesn't have fears? – but I take less crap and don't dwell on what people think about me, unless they are my nearest and dearest. I don't bear grudges. One therapist told me he felt I had 'post-traumatic growth', which makes sense, and I rather like the sound of it.

I bounce.

During my 'down years', I missed the explosion of social media. It took me a while to get used to the confrontations of anonymous keyboard warriors and to learn the value of not bashing out a retort I later regret. I've been 'burned' a couple of times. Mostly, I now leave those situations. And I love Facebook. My teenage kids repeatedly ask me if I think 'I have a problem'.

A 21st-century addiction, I guess. Or should I say 'dependency'? (Winks.)

So, what the hell happened to me? And why did I get better?

For every expert I have asked – the professionals (on sleep) and the personal friends (on me) – there is a different theory.

Some have argued I suffered PTSD on the end of my marriage, or that I was depressed before I stopped sleeping, i.e. my insomnia was a result of mental health issues, rather than the other way around.

With both of these notions – especially the second – I have issues. Depression doesn't come on overnight: I was fine on 15th July. When I received that bad news from my then-husband on 16th July, I was not. And is the end of a marriage a trauma? Maybe, for me, it was.

Dr Sami Timimi's suggestion that I had an 'ordinary' and 'understandable' reaction to a distressing life event makes sense (see page 98). He posits that my insomnia then became the issue. I turned the problem into *the problem*. Then there is Professor Guy Leschziner's take that sleep is a 'result of a multitude of factors: the physiological, the neurological, the psychological and the environmental' (see page 191). This also speaks to me. I needed a total change in all of those factors to begin my recovery.

I didn't just pick up the pieces. I also found new ones to build with.

And then there are the pills, specifically the benzos. My own verdict is that I was put on these drugs too easily, given too many of them for too long. Then it became a mess. Rehab was a disaster because of a lack of understanding about my particular problem. The clinic team started to pull me off the benzos too quickly. I then finished the job myself – with a way-too-rapid reduction.

I'm almost certain I suffered from 'post-withdrawal syndrome', briefly defined by Professor Heather Ashton as 'an amalgam of pharmacological and psychological factors directly and indirectly related to benzodiazepine use'. Professor Joanna Moncrieff is really good on this in her book, *Psychiatric Drugs*, some of which I quote on page 143. As is Melanie Davis of REST (page 130).

Ultimately, of course, I will never know the answer to either of these questions. The major task now is to stop this happening again. And I'm not sure that I could. It's not as if I made any obvious mistakes that I can learn from – except maybe not ever to take another benzodiazepine. It may be staying on anti-depressants will offer me some protection. But I was already on trazodone (albeit a mild dose) when the Crash hit me. And I then took the drug for years at a far higher dose, with no discernible effect.

My recovery started more *despite* the drugs I was taking, rather than because of them.

Three things I would say did help me:

1. 'Entry-level' advice on diet and exercise. This may sound obvious but it's all about the application, rather than saying 'yes, yes, yes' at the theory and carrying on with the same old habits. If you eat well and move around more, there is no question it will improve your mood and give you more energy during the day. Both of which lead to better sleep.

2. If I had to name a 'product', I would say invest in a weighted blanket (see page 228). It definitely helps me a) keep warm and b) sleep more deeply in the autumn and winter months.

3. The CBTi rules. The night before writing this concluding passage, I had a broken night's sleep. It could be that I knew I was approaching the end of this book and was quite 'wired'. Or maybe because, emboldened by my achievement, I had also jumped down on my pregabalin several milligrams and – hurray! – insomnia is one side effect of my taper.

   It took me till 2am to fall asleep. I had a bad dream and woke up at 3.30am. I could have panicked and or/despaired. But I didn't. I went downstairs and made myself a hot drink, brought it to bed and picked up a book. 'Don't turn the problem into *the problem*,' I said it out loud, in the dead of night. (Thanks, Dr Sami.)

As Dr Sophie Bostock would have it, my sleep
pressure built up, I got tired again – and I almost
fought against this because I was enjoying my
book so much. However, at 4am I did lie down. I
slept till 5.30am, and then again until 7am. Four
and a half hours: within the Four-Hour Rule.

Overall, I would say I am more emotionally resilient than
I was back in year one. Although the sudden end of a
marriage – the catalyst for all this – was a pretty big thing,
you have to admit. But this does not mean I'm going to
stop myself open-heartedly loving someone for fear this
might happen again. I also have close emotional connections with many people, not just a romantic partner.
Heartbreak is part of life.

I am loving each day and the little pleasures it brings.
Sure, disaster may lurk around every corner – and didn't
the wider world see enough of that in the early 2020s?
Things could go crashing down again. But maybe there is
a tiny chance they will not.

Some lines I find helpful if I find myself slipping:

From Baz Luhrmann's *Strictly Ballroom*: A life lived in
fear is a life half lived.

From Rainer Maria Rilke: Just keep going / No feeling
is final.

From Professor Chris Whitty, thrust to fame during
the COVID pandemic: Next slide, please.

Slightly bastardized from the 12-Step programme: Just
for today: I am doing bloody well.

And from me: On we go!

13th January 2021

7 HOURS, 20 MINUTES (A CHUNK OF 6 HOURS, AND A
SCHLUFF OF 80 MINUTES)

I have hit my magic number.

I squint at the clock, raise a sleepy eyebrow in surprise
and joy. I ask Alexa to play Radio 4. As soporific old
Dominic starts to bang on about the business news, I turn
over, bunch the duvet around me, and fall back to sleep.

Acknowledgements

Here's a curtain call for the people who supported me, tolerated me, tried to keep me going or helped me get started again... or basically just kept me alive:

First my wonderful family: Lawrence Levy (Dad), Drs Sarah and Miles Levy, Ben and Sophie; my amazing kids: you know who you are. Aunty Valerie; Hania and Joel Cooper, and family.

JK, you also know who you are.

Friends I'll put alphabetically, because there is no way I can make a 'hierarchy' (MASSIVE apologies if I've left anyone out): Katalin Aradi, Justine Berkovitz, Lucie Chaumeton, Winnie Dhaliwal, Sean Guinness, Leah Hardy, Hermione Ireland, Rachel Morris, Alex Oldroyd, Becky Sheaves, Sam Sheril.

'Worky' people: Tania Minkoff Allen, Kathryn Blundell, Rimi Atwal, Ellie Hughes, Jo Morrell and the 'TeleGrazians': Jane Bruton, Lucy Dunn, Vicki Harper, Marianne Jones. The ladies from 'No 1', who helped me with my first feature 'back' and the idea for a blog, which led to a column which led to a book: Helen Carroll, Helen Foster, Kathryn Knight.

Dr Hadi Zambarakji for saving my sight, Dr Kassim, Michele, and Dr Sinha, Anthony Stone for (trying to) save my mind, and becoming a great friend, Karen Levison for being tough and sunny, and taking my punches.

When it comes to *The Insomnia Diaries*, I'd first like to thank my school English teacher Mr Jones, my inspiration, and first crush. TRJC, you set me up for a life of enjoying reading and writing. Then, Julie Burchill for encouragement, lunch, and a ride up the Brighton BA i360 Tower, Dr Matt Morgan for (as well as saving many lives) introducing me to his agent, the wonderful Charlotte Seymour, who continued to have faith in this book. For support and inspiration, Marian Keyes and Tony Baines. Sophie Bostock for the foreword, much advice, and the 'passive water-based body heating' – and all the contributing experts named upfront for their wisdom and experience.

Also to Stephanie Jackson at Octopus for taking me on with your terrific team: Ella Parsons, Juliette Norsworthy, Megan Brown, Hazel O'Brien, Kevin Hawkins and his team, and Caroline Alberti.

A special final mention to Bret and Jemaine, and Xander and Richard.

Endnotes

All websites accessed February 2021.

Foreword

Espie, C. A., Emsley, R., Kyle, S. D., Gordon, C., Drake, C. L., Siriwardena, A. N., ... & Luik, A. I. (2019). Effect of digital cognitive behavioral therapy for insomnia on health, psychological well-being, and sleep-related quality of life: A randomized clinical trial. *JAMA Psychiatry*, 76(1), 21–30.

Longstreth, W. T. J., Koepsell, T. D., Ton, T. G., Hendrickson, A. F., & van Belle, G. (2007). The epidemiology of narcolepsy. *Sleep*, 30(1), 13–26.

Morin, C. M., & Benca, R. (Mar. 2012). Chronic insomnia. *Lancet*, 379(9821), 1129–1141.

Pigeon, W. R., Bishop, T. M., & Krueger, K. M. (2017). Insomnia as a precipitating factor in new onset mental illness: A Systematic review of recent findings. *Current Psychiatry Reports*, 19(8), 44.

PART ONE: DARKNESS DESCENDS

Page 20, What is insomnia?

Dr Sophie Bostock, interview with author, November 2020.

Healthline (24 Jul. 2020). Everything you need to know about insomnia. Retrieved from www.healthline.com/health/insomnia

Lubit, R. H. (21 Aug. 2019). Sleep–wake disorders clinical presentation. *Medscape*.

Mayo Clinic (15 Oct. 2016). Insomnia. Retrieved from www.mayoclinic.org/diseases-conditions/insomnia/symptoms-causes/syc-20355167

Roth, T. (2007). Insomnia: Definition, prevalence, etiology, and consequences. *Journal of Clinical Sleep Medicine*, 3(5 suppl), S7–S10.

Saddichha, S. (2010). Diagnosis and treatment of chronic insomnia. *Annals of Indian Academy of Neurology*, 13(2), 94–102.

Sleep Foundation (4 Sep. 2020). Insomnia. Retrieved from www.sleepfoundation.org/insomnia

Sleep Foundation (22 Jan. 2021). Women and sleep. Retrieved from www.sleepfoundation.org/women-sleep

Page 24, Your first sleepless stop: your GP

Dr Sarah Levy, interview with author, June 2020.

Page 27, 21st July, sleep hygiene

Sleep Foundation (14 Aug. 2020). Sleep hygiene. Retrieved from www.sleepfoundation.org/sleep-hygiene

Sleep.org. What is sleep hygiene. Retrieved from www.sleep.org/sleep-hygiene

UT News (19 Jul. 2019). Take a warm bath 1–2 hours before bedtime to get better sleep, researchers find. Retrieved from www.news.utexas.edu/2019/07/19/take-a-warm-bath-1-2-hours-before-bedtime-to-get-better-sleep-researchers-find/

Page 29, Sleeping pills, anti-depressants and other 'sleep aids'

Barnard, K., Peveler, R. C., & Holt, R. I. (2013). Antidepressant medication as a risk factor for type 2 diabetes and impaired glucose regulation: Systematic review. *Diabetes Care*, 36(10), 3337–3345.

Dr Sophie Bostock, interview with author, September 2020.

Fiore, V. (11 Sep. 2020). Antidepressants dispensed up almost a quarter in last five years. Chemist + Druggist. Retrieved from www.chemistanddruggist.co.uk/news/antidepressants-dispensed-almost-quarter-last-five-years

Grigg-Damberger, M. M., & Ianakieva, D. (2017). Poor quality control of over-the-counter melatonin: What they say is often not what you get. *Journal of Clinical Sleep Medicine*, *13*(2), 163–165.

Harvard Health Publishing (2019). Improving sleep: A guide to a good night's rest. A Harvard Medical School Special Health Report, 24–27.

Healthline (25 Feb. 2020). Why withdrawal symptoms can be serious when someone stops taking antidepressants. Retrieved from www.healthline.com/health-news/antidepressants-physical-dependence-withdrawal-symptoms

Kirsch, I. (2014). Antidepressants and the placebo effect. *Zeitschrift für Psychologie*, *222*(3), 128–134.

Mind (Aug. 2016). Sleeping pills and minor tranquillisers. Retrieved from www.mind.org.uk/information-support/drugs-and-treatments/sleeping-pills-and-minor-tranquillisers/about-sleeping-pills-and-minor-tranquillisers/

National Institute for Health and Care Excellence (15 Jan. 2015). Hypnotics. Retrieved from www.nice.org.uk/advice/ktt6/resources/hypnotics-pdf-1632173521093

Public Health England (3 Dec. 2020). Prescribed medicines review: Summary. Retrieved from www.gov.uk/government/publications/prescribed-medicines-review-report/prescribed-medicines-review-summary

Page 35, 23rd July

Diamond, J. (2001). *Snake Oil and Other Preoccupations*. Vintage.

Preston, P. (1 Jul. 2001). Polished Diamond. *The Observer*. Retrieved from www.theguardian.com/theobserver/2001/jul/01/society

Page 39, How much sleep do you really need and when should you get it?

American Psychological Association (May 2020). Why sleep is important. Retrieved from www.apa.org/topics/sleep/why

Dr Sophie Bostock, interview with the author, July 2019.

Capuccio, F. P., D'Elia, L., Strazzullo, P., & Miller, M. A. (2010). Sleep duration and all-cause mortality: A systematic review and meta-analysis of prospective studies. *Sleep*, *33*(5), 585–592.

Centers for Disease Control and Prevention (2017). How much sleep do I need? Retrieved from www.cdc.gov/sleep/about_sleep/how_much_sleep.html

Consensus Conference Panel, Watson, N. F., Badr, M. S., Belenky, G., Bliwise, D. L., Buxton, O. M., ... & Tasali, E. (2015). Recommended amount of sleep for a healthy adult: A joint consensus statement of the American Academy of Sleep Medicine and Sleep Research Society. *Journal of Clinical Sleep Medicine*, *11*(6), 591–592.

Harvard Health Publishing (Aug. 2019). How much sleep do we really need? Retrieved from www.health.harvard.edu/staying-healthy/how-much-sleep-do-we-really-need

Sleep Foundation (31 Jul. 2020). How much sleep do we really need? Retrieved from www.sleepfoundation.org/how-sleep-works/how-much-sleep-do-we-really-need

University of Warwick (May 2010). Short sleep increases risk of death & over long sleep can indicate serious illness. Retrieved from www.warwick.ac.uk/newsandevents/pressreleases/short_sleep_increases/

Page 46, When you are likely to be referred to a psychiatrist and what might happen

Mind. Drugs and treatments. Retrieved from www.mind.org.uk/information-support/drugs-and-treatments/

Mind (2016). Psychiatric medication: Drug names A–Z. Retrieved from www.mind.org.uk/information-support/drugs-and-treatments/medication/drug-names-a-z/

Mind (2016). Psychiatric medication: What is psychiatric medication? Retrieved from www.mind.org.uk/information-support/drugs-and-treatments/medication/about-medication/

Dr Sami Timimi, interview with author, June 2020.

Page 53, What makes someone go from temporarily sleepless to a full-blown chronic insomniac?

Dr Sophie Bostock, interview with author, December 2020.

PART TWO: TOSSING AND TURNING

Page 60, Eat more carbs, eat fewer carbs

Afaghi, A., O'Connor, H., & Chow, C. M. (2007). High-glycemic-index carbohydrate meals shorten sleep onset. *The American Journal of Clinical Nutrition*, *85*(2), 426–430.

Gangwisch, J. E., Hale, L., St-Onge, M. P., Choi, L., LeBlanc, E. S., Malaspina, D., ... & Lane, D. (2020). High glycemic index and glycemic load diets as risk factors for insomnia: Analyses from the Women's Health Initiative. *The American Journal of Clinical Nutrition*, *111*(2), 429–439.

Page 60, Try cognitive behavioural therapy

NHS (16 Jul. 2019). Overview: Cognitive behavioural therapy (CBT). Retrieved from www.nhs.uk/conditions/cognitive-behavioural-therapy-cbt/

Page 66, What to do if you feel suicidal

Mind (2020). Suicidal feelings. Retrieved from www.mind.org.uk/media-a/6164/suicidal-feelings-2020.pdf

Rilke, R. M. (1996). Go to the limits of your longing. In: Macy, J., & Barrows, A. (trans.). *Rilke's Book of Hours: Love Poems to God*. Riverhead Books.

Page 80, Insomnia: how it affects your physical health

Dr Sophie Bostock, interview with author, July 2010.

Harvard Health Publishing (2019). Improving sleep: A guide to a good night's rest. A Harvard Medical School Special Health Report.

Kim, H., Hegde, S., LaFiura, C., et al. (2021). COVID-19 illness in relation to sleep and burnout. *BMJ Nutrition, Prevention & Health*

Page 90, 9th February

Dr Sarah Levy, interview with author, August 2020.

Lubit, R. H. (5 Nov. 2018). What are the DSM-5 diagnostic criteria for borderline personality disorder (BDP)? *Medscape*.

Page 94, Personality disorders

American Psychiatric Association (Nov. 2018). What are personality disorders? Retrieved from www.psychiatry.org/patients-families/personality-disorders/what-are-personality-disorders

Dr Sophie Bostock, interview with author, September 2020.

Freedenthal, S. (15 Oct. 2013). Should we abolish the diagnosis of borderline personality? [blog]. GoodTherapy. Retrieved from www.goodtherapy.org/blog/should-we-abolish-the-diagnosis-of-borderline-personality-1015134

Mayo Clinic (23 Sep. 2016). Personality disorders. Retrieved from www.mayoclinic.org/diseases-conditions/personality-disorders/symptoms-causes/syc-20354463

NHS (12 Oct. 2020). Personality disorder. Retrieved from www.nhs.uk/conditions/personality-disorder/

Rethink Mental Illness. Personality disorders. Retrieved from www.rethink.org/advice-and-information/about-mental-illness/learn-more-about-conditions/personality-disorders/

Dr Sami Timimi, interview with author, August 2020.

Page 103, On Heather Ashton and *The Ashton Manual*

Ashton, C. H. (Aug. 2002). *Benzodiazepines: How They Work and How to Withdraw* (aka *The Ashton Manual*). Retrieved from www.benzo.org.uk/manual/bzcha00.htm

www.benzo.org.uk

Page 104, But, life gets worse when you try to come off the bloody benzos...

Moncrieff, J. (2020). *A Straight Talking Introduction to Psychiatric Drugs: The Truth About How They Work and How to Come Off Them* [second edition]. PCCS Books, 147.

Page 106, Addicted or dependent? The politics

Addiction Center (30 Nov. 2020). Addiction vs. dependence. Retrieved from www.addictioncenter.com/addiction/addiction-vs-dependence/

Dr Mark Horowitz, interview with author, March 2021.

Page 117, The 12-Step programme

Alcoholics Anonymous. The Twelve Steps of Alcoholics Anonymous. Retrieved from www.alcoholics-anonymous.org.uk/about-aa/the-12-steps-of-aa

Nicky Walton-Flynn, interview with author, July 2020.

Wilson, W. G. (1939). *Alcoholics Anonymous: The Story of How More Than One Hundred Men Have Recovered from Alcoholism*. The Anonymous Press.

Page 129, Rehab – where did it all go wrong?

Nicky Walton-Flynn, interview with author, July 2020.

Page 130, Coming off benzos: what *should* happen?

Melanie Davis, interview with author, July 2020.

Page 143, Year Ten: A note from the future

Moncrieff, J. (2020). *A Straight Talking Introduction to Psychiatric Drugs: The Truth About How They Work and How to Come Off Them* [second edition]. PCCS Books, 147.

Page 145, 14th January

Letter to author and her GP from private psychiatrist.

Page 146, The definition of psychosis

NHS (10 Dec. 2019). Overview: Psychosis. Retrieved from www.nhs.uk/conditions/psychosis/

Dr Sami Timimi, interview with author, August 2020.

Page 151, 3rd March

Letter to author and her GP from private psychiatrist.

Page 161, On sleep trackers

Glazer Baron, K., Abbott, S., Jao, N., Manalo, N., & Mullen, R. (2017). Orthosomnia: Are some patients taking the quantified self too far? *Journal of Clinical Sleep Medicine*, *13*(2), 351–354.

Professor Guy Leschziner, interview with author, August 2019.

Page 165, 23rd January

Letter to author and her GP from NHS psychiatrist.

Page 166, Says Dr Sami Timimi from the future

Dr Sami Timimi, interview with author, August 2020.

Page 168, 15th June

Letter to author and her GP from NHS psychiatrist.

Page 169, 6th June

Letter to author and her GP from NHS psychiatrist.

Page 176, The anatomy of sleep

National Institute of Neurological Disorders and Stroke (13 Aug. 2019). Brain basics: Understanding sleep. Retrieved from www.ninds.nih.gov/Disorders/Patient-Caregiver-Education/Understanding-Sleep

Schneider, L. (2017). Anatomy and physiology of normal sleep. In: Miglis, M. G. (ed.). *Sleep and Neurologic Disease*. Academic Press, 1–28.

Page 182, 14th December

Letter to author and her GP from sleep specialist.

PART THREE: OPENING THE CURTAINS

Page 189, Paradoxical insomnia, or sleep state misperception

Professor Guy Leschziner, interview with author, September 2020.

Wikipedia (12 Jan. 2021). Sleep state misperception. Retrieved from https://en.wikipedia.org/wiki/Sleep_state_misperception

Page 192, 19th December

Letter to author and her GP from NHS psychiatrist.

Page 204, 22nd May

Levy, M. (22 May 2019). Insomnia robbed me of my job, family, and sanity. *Daily Mail*. Retrieved from www.dailymail.co.uk/femail/article-7059837/Insomnia-robbed-job-family-sanity-former-editor-Mother-Baby-magazine.html

Page 205, 25th May

Fortune Business Insights (Aug. 2020). Fitness tracker market size, share & COVID-19 impact analysis. Retrieved from www.fortunebusinessinsights.com/toc/fitness-tracker-market-103358

McGurk, S. (31 Mar. 2020). The business of sleep. *GQ Magazine*. Retrieved from www.gq-magazine.co.uk/lifestyle/article/the-business-of-sleep

RAND Europe (30 Nov. 2016). Lack of sleep costing UK economy up to £40 billion a year. Retrieved from www.rand.org/news/press/2016/11/30/index1.html

Page 207, 5th June

Letter to author and her GP from NHS psychiatrist.

Page 209, So what is pregabalin?

Green, K., O'Dowd, N. C., Watt, H., Majeed, A., & Pinder, R. J. (2019). Prescribing trends of gabapentin, pregabalin, and oxycodone: A secondary analysis of primary care prescribing patterns in England. *BJGP Open*, *3*(3).

Professor David Healy, interview with author, September 2019.

Page 211, 18th June

Levy, M. (18 Jun. 2019). I've just woken up from a seven-year news coma – what have I missed? *Daily Telegraph*. Retrieved from www.telegraph.co.uk/women/life/just-woken-seven-year-news-coma-have-missed/

Page 215, Cognitive behavioural therapy for insomnia (CBTi)

Dr Sophie Bostock, interview with author, September 2020.

Drake, C., Roehrs, T., Shambroom, J., & Roth, T. (2013). Caffeine effects on sleep taken 0, 3, or 6 hours before going to bed. *Journal of Clinical Sleep Medicine*, *9*(11), 1195–1200.

Sleepio. CBT for insomnia – the science behind Sleepio. Retrieved from www.sleepio.com/cbt-for-insomnia/

www.thesleepscientist.com/

Page 219, 11th July

Burchill, J. (7 Jun. 2020). Psychedelic dreams are the best thing about lockdown. *Telegraph*. Retrieved from www.telegraph.co.uk/news/2020/06/07/psychedelic-dreams-best-thing-lockdown/

Page 219, Early bird or night owl? What is your 'chronotype'?

Dr Sophie Bostock, interview with author, August 2019.

Curtis, B. J., Ashbrook, L. H., Young, T., Finn, L. A., Fu, Y. H., Ptáček, L. J., & Jones, C. R. (2019). Extreme morning chronotypes are often familial and not exceedingly rare: The estimated prevalence of advanced sleep phase, familial advanced sleep phase, and advanced sleep–wake phase disorder in a sleep clinic population. *Sleep*, 42(10), zsz148.

MasterClass (2 Feb. 2021). How to determine your chronotype and ideal sleep schedule. Retrieved from www.masterclass.com/articles/how-to-determine-your-chronotype

Sleep Foundation (8 Jan. 2021). Chronotypes. Retrieved from www.sleepfoundation.org/how-sleep-works/chronotypes

University of Birmingham (10 Jun. 2019). Night owls can 'retrain' their body clocks to improve mental well-being and performance. ScienceDaily. Retrieved from www.sciencedaily.com/releases/2019/06/190610100622.htm

Page 225, Why lack of sleep turns you into a toddler who missed a nap

Susan Quilliam, interview with author, September 2019.

Page 230, Cannabidiol (CBD)

Harvard Health Publishing (24 Aug. 2018). Cannabidiol (CBD) – what we know and what we don't. Retrieved from www.health.harvard.edu/blog/cannabidiol-cbd-what-we-know-and-what-we-dont-2018082414476

Heathline (11 May 2020). CBD for insomnia: Benefits, side effects, and treatment. Retrieved from www.healthline.com/health/cbd-for-insomnia

Medical News Today (29 Sept. 2020). Does CBD help treat insomnia? Retrieved from www.medicalnewstoday.com/articles/cbd-for-insomnia

Shannon, S., Lewis, N., Lee, H., & Hughes, S. (2019). Cannabidiol in anxiety and sleep: A large case series. *The Permanente Journal*, *23*, 18–41.

Page 231, A quick note on bedding

Professor Adam Fox, interview with author, August 2019.

James O'Loan, interview with author, August 2019.

Warren, J. (26 Apr. 2019). Clostridiales, Neisseriales, and Fusobacteriales: The bacteria that lurks in four-week-old bedsheets. Time4Sleep. Retrieved from www.time4sleep.co.uk/blog/clostridiales-neisseriales-and-fusobacteriales-the-bacteria-that-lurks-in-four-week-old-bedsheets

Warren, J. (28 Feb. 2020). How often should you change your bed sheets. Time4Sleep. Retrieved from www.time4sleep.co.uk/blog/how-often-should-you-change-your-bed-sheets

Page 238, 25th August

Dr Sophie Bostock, interview with author, July 2019.

Breus, M. (23 Jul. 2019). 7 ways to sleep better in the next heatwave. The Sleep Doctor. Retrieved from www.thesleepdoctor.com/2019/07/23/sleep-better-next-heat-wave/

Department of Health, Government of Australia. Sleeping in very hot weather. Retrieved from www.healthywa.wa.gov. au/Articles/S_T/Sleeping-in-very-hot-weather

Medical News Today (14 Mar. 2020). What happens if you drink too much water? Retrieved from www.medicalnewstoday. com/articles/318619

Somerset Urology Associates (26 Oct. 2013). Drink three litres of water a day or risk kidney stones warns expert as hospital admissions for renal conditions rise. Retrieved from www.somerseturology.co.uk/food-tips/ water-a-day-or-risk-kidney-stones/

Page 240, Sleeping in winter

Dr Sophie Bostock, interview with author, November 2020.

Breus, M. (9 Dec. 2019). Why is my insomnia worse in winter? Your cold-weather sleep questions answered. The Sleep Doctor. Retrieved from www.thesleepdoctor. com/2019/12/09/why-is-my-insomnia-worse-in-winter-your-cold-weather-sleep-questions-answered/

Haghayegh, S., Khoshnevis, S., Smolensky, M. H., Diller, K. R., & Castriotta, R. J. (2019). Before-bedtime passive body heating by warm shower or bath to improve sleep: A systematic review and meta-analysis. *Sleep Medicine Review Aug*(46), 124–135.

Page 243, What you can learn about sleep from a long-haul pilot

Dr Sophie Bostock, interview with author, October 2019.

Captain Charles Everett, interview with author, October 2019.

AFTERWORD

Page 256, Is there a science behind our dreams?

Professor Guy Leschziner, interview with author, April 2020.

Page 258, Common dreams: what do they mean?

Atherton, S. The 10 most common dreams & what they mean. Dreams. Retrieved from www.dreams.co.uk/sleep-matters-club/the-10-most-common-dreams-what-they-mean/

Professor Guy Leschziner, interview with author, April 2020.

Page 262, So, what the hell happened to me? And why did I get better?

Ashton, C. H. (2004). Protracted withdrawal symptoms from benzodiazepines. Retrieved from www.benzo.org.uk/pws04.htm

Further Reading & Resources

Books

Professor David Healy, *Psychiatric Drugs Explained*, London: Churchill Livingstone, 2016

Professor Guy Leschziner, *The Nocturnal Brain: Nightmares, Neuroscience and the Secret World of Sleep*, London: Simon & Schuster, 2019

Dr Guy Meadows, *The Sleep Book: How to Sleep Well Every Night*, London: Orion, 2014

Professor Joanna Moncrieff, *A Straight Talking Introduction to Psychiatric Drugs: The Truth About How They Work and How to Come Off Them*, second edition, Monmouth: PCCS Books, 2020

Dr Sami Timimi, *Insane Medicine: How the Mental Health Industry Creates Damaging Treatment Traps and How You Can Escape Them,* self-published, 2021

Matthew Walker, *Why We Sleep: The New Science of Sleep and Dreams*, London: Penguin, 2018

Useful Websites and Resources

Note: If you live outside the UK, speak to your doctor about where to seek help and they should be able to direct you to the appropriate resources.

samaritans.org
   Call the Samaritans on 116 123

giveusashout.org
   text 'SHOUT' to 85258

mind.org.uk

Alcoholics Anonymous: alcoholics-anonymous.org.uk

Allergy UK: allergyuk.co.uk

American Psychiatric Association: psychiatry.org

benzo.org.uk

benzobuddies.org/forum

Bristol & District Tranquilliser Project: btpinfo.org.uk

www.changegrowlive.org
   www.changegrowlive.org/recovery-experience-sleeping-
   pills-and-tranquillisers-rest
   www.changegrowlive.org/advice-info/alcohol-drugs/
   drugs-chat-to-someone-online

Council for Information on Tranquillisers, Antidepressants,
   and Painkillers: citap.org.uk

DermaSilk: dermasilk.co.uk

Mad In America: madinamerica.com

Mayo Clinic: mayoclinic.org

Narcotics Anonymous: ukna.org

nhs.uk

Rethink Mental Illness: rethink.org

Sleepio: sleepio.co.uk

Dr Sophie Bostock: thesleepscientist.com
Dr Michael Breus: thesleepdoctor.com

The Academy of Experts

Dr Sophie Bostock studied medicine at the University of Nottingham, followed by an MSc in Entrepreneurship and a Ph.D in Health Psychology at University College London (UCL). She successfully helped to make the CBTi Sleepio programme available on the NHS to a fifth of the UK population. Sophie has delivered talks for TEDx and Talks at Google, and regularly features as a sleep expert in national media.

Melanie Davis is the manager of REST (Recovery, Experience, Sleeping Pills and Tranquilisers) – a support service for people who take sleeping pills and benzodiazepines. She is also a member of the Council for Evidence-Based Psychiatry and sits on the All-Party Parliamentary Group for Prescribed Drug Dependence. Melanie has offered emotional and practical support to more than 3,000 adults who are dependent on prescription medication.

Dr Mark Horowitz is a training psychiatrist and research fellow in the UCL Department of Psychiatry. He is originally from Sydney, Australia. In 2015, Mark completed a PhD in the neurobiological effects of antidepressants at the Institute of Psychiatry, Psychology and Neuroscience at King's College London. He has an interest in rational prescribing in psychiatry, including de-prescribing – when and how to stop medications. He is currently a Clinical Research Fellow on the RADAR trial and co-authored the Royal College of Psychiatry guidelines on how to stop antidepressants.

Professor Guy Leschziner is professor of neurology and sleep medicine at King's College London and leads the Sleep Disorders Centre at Guy's Hospital, one of Europe's leading sleep services. He is the author of *The Nocturnal Brain: Nightmares, Neuroscience and the Secret World of Sleep*, and is the presenter of BBC Radio 4's 'Mysteries of Sleep'.

Professor Joanna Moncrieff studied medicine at Newcastle University, then trained in psychiatry in London and the south east. She spent a decade as a consultant for a psychiatric rehabilitation inpatient unit, and for the last three years she has been based in community mental health services in north-east London. Joanna teaches and researches at University College London (UCL) and is a founder and co-chair of the Critical Psychiatry Network.

Susan Quilliam is a psychologist, relationship coach, author and agony aunt. She is a professional associate of the College of Sexual and Relationship Therapists, and an associate member of the Royal Society of Medicine. Susan also works as an ambassador for Relate Cambridge and is a patron of the Outsiders charity.

Anthony Stone has been a psychotherapist in private practice for more than 30 years, after a prior career in business. His orientation is existential and humanistic, and he is psychoanalytically informed. Anthony is sceptical about the efficacy of medication and believes that no one should become a psychotherapist until they are at least 70 years old: it's a job for an 'elder'.

Dr Sami Timimi is a consultant child and adolescent psychiatrist and visiting professor of Child Psychiatry and Mental Health Improvement who lives and works in Lincolnshire. He also writes on mental health from a critical perspective, and has been published on subjects including childhood, psychotherapy and behavioural problems. Sami's latest book is *Insane Medicine: How the Mental Health Industry Creates Damaging Treatment Traps and How You Can Escape Them.*

Nicky Walton-Flynn is an addiction psychologist and trauma therapist. In 2007, she founded Addiction Therapy London. Nicky has worked at a private residential rehab in London, as well as with charity organizations offering harm minimization interventions for homeless people and street addicts.

Index

About the Author

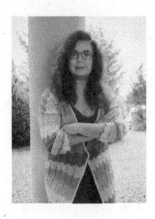

Miranda Levy is a journalist and author with more than 25 years' experience. Starting out on magazines including *Cosmopolitan* and *New Woman* (RIP), she then hacked it at the *Daily Mail* and *Sunday Mirror* before heading back to glossies and the launches of *Glamour* and *Grazia*. She had two babies, wrote *The Rough Guide to Babies* in 2006, and became editor of *Mother & Baby*, where she was twice nominated for a British Society of Magazine Editors award. Now a freelance writer and editor for national newspapers, she covers many topics – but particularly health – for titles including the *Telegraph* platforms, the *Mail on Sunday* and the *i*. Miranda has contributed to the *Spectator*, the *Jewish Chronicle* and the *New York Post*.

talesofaninsomniac.com
mirandalevy.co.uk
Twitter: @mirandalevycopy